A Foot in the Door™

INTERNSHIP & VOLUNTEER OPPORTUNITIES

for People Who Love Movement

Susan Dobinick

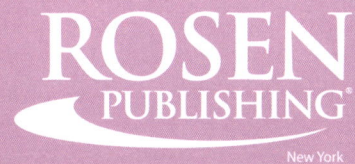
Rosen Publishing
New York

Published in 2013 by The Rosen Publishing Group, Inc.
29 East 21st Street, New York, NY 10010

Copyright © 2013 by The Rosen Publishing Group, Inc.

First Edition

All rights reserved. No part of this book may be reproduced in any form without permission in writing from the publisher, except by a reviewer.

Library of Congress Cataloging-in-Publication Data

Dobinick, Susan.
Internship & volunteer opportunities for people who love movement /Susan Dobinick.
    p. cm.—(A foot in the door)
Includes bibliographical references and index.
ISBN 978-1-4488-8298-4 (library binding)
1. Dance—Vocational guidance. 2. Dance—Study and teaching (Internship) 3. Voluntarism. I. Title.
GV1597.D63 2013
793.3023—dc23

                                              2012017553

Manufactured in the United States of America

CPSIA Compliance Information: Batch #W13YA: For further information, contact Rosen Publishing, New York, New York, at 1-800-237-9932.

Contents

Introduction	5
Chapter One RESEARCHING YOUR OUTDOOR INTERESTS	8
Chapter Two FINDING OPPORTUNITIES	20
Chapter Three COACHING	32
Chapter Four TEACHING	37
Chapter Five WORKING WITH INDIVIDUALS	45
Chapter Six PERFORMING ARTS	52
Chapter Seven TOURISM AND RECREATION	57
Chapter Eight MAKING THE MOST OF YOUR EXPERIENCE	65
Glossary	72
For More Information	74
For Further Reading	76
Bibliography	77
Index	78

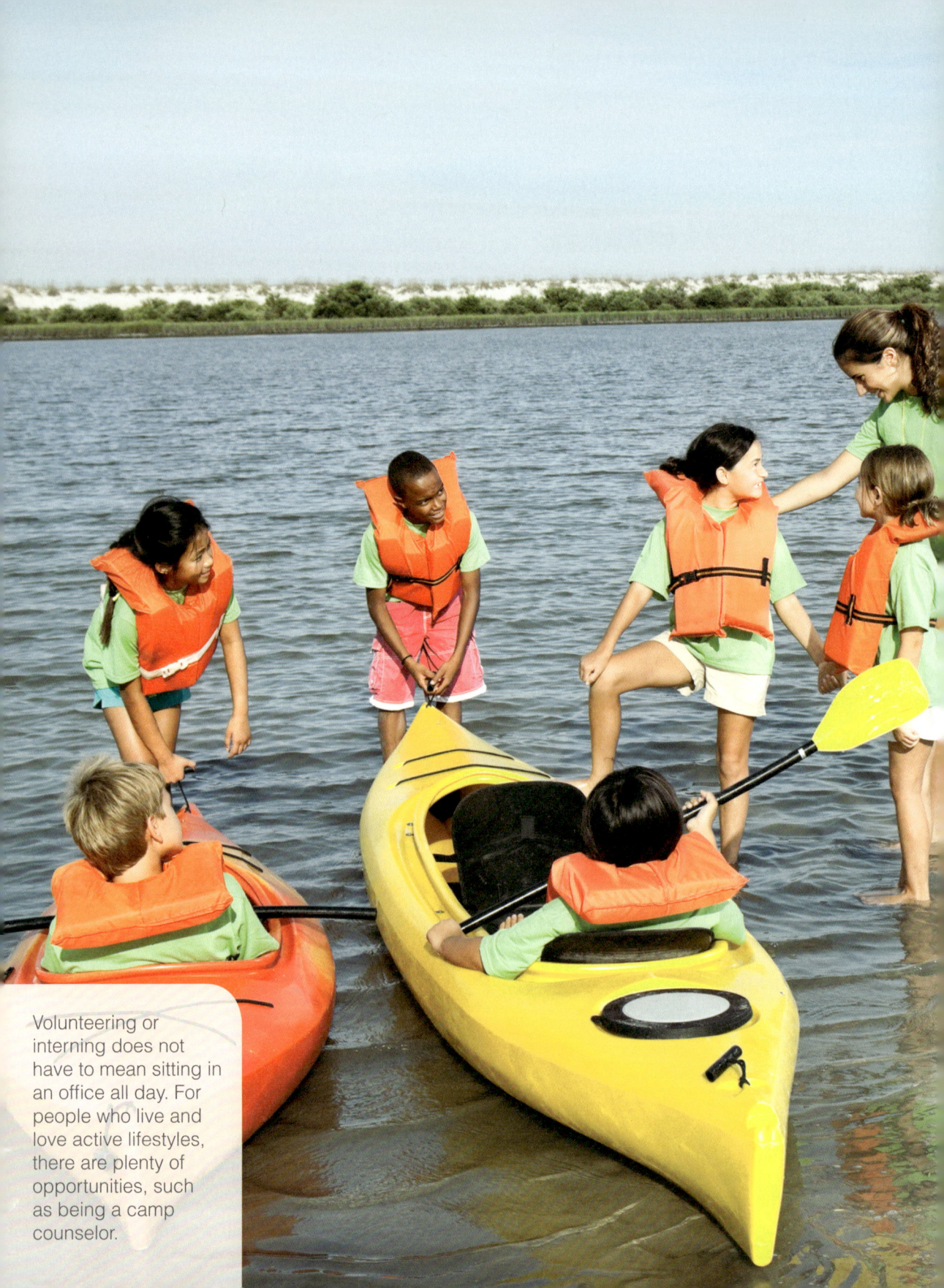

Volunteering or interning does not have to mean sitting in an office all day. For people who live and love active lifestyles, there are plenty of opportunities, such as being a camp counselor.

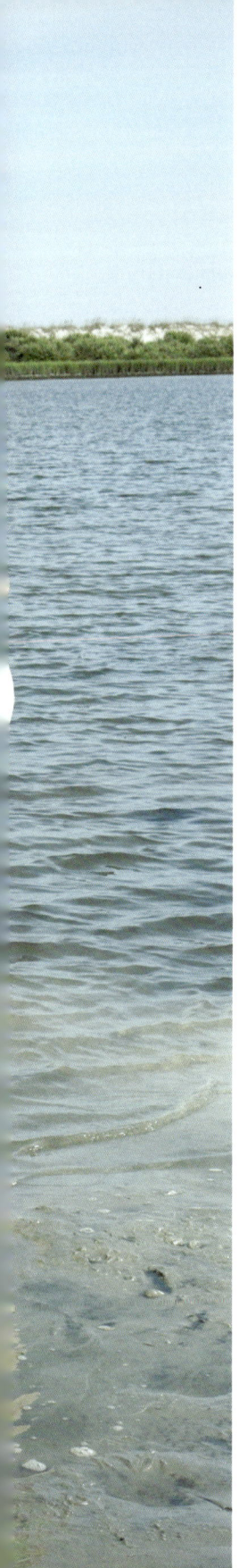

Introduction

For many young people, after-school jobs are a part of everyday life. But it can be hard to find a job in the field you are interested in pursuing as a career. Often these types of jobs are offered only to people with more education or experience than most young people have. But this does not mean there is not a way to explore your career interests as a young person. Volunteer and internship opportunities are a great way to find out more about what it means to work in a particular field. For people who love sports and staying active, volunteering or interning at the right organization or company can show them how a hobby can become a career.

Volunteering means offering to help out without getting paid. Volunteer opportunities mostly occur at nonprofit organizations, or groups that do not make money from the work they do. People choose to volunteer for many reasons. It is a way of helping a cause that someone cares about. It can

internship & volunteer opportunities for people who love movement

demonstrate to colleges that applicants have a sense of civic responsibility and care about their community. It can also give valuable experience that will help a person find further career opportunities later on.

Volunteer opportunities can be casual or more structured, depending on the organization. Some organizations have long-standing volunteer programs with specific duties and goals, like coordinating an event or coaching a team through an entire season. Others, especially smaller organizations, may just need an extra hand to help out with tasks as they arise.

An internship is a form of job training that is similar to being an entry-level apprentice in a field. Interns can be paid or unpaid, and interns can work at nonprofit organizations or for-profit companies. Like volunteer experiences, these can be structured or casual. People often choose to intern so that they can understand how a particular type of business or organization works from the inside. Interning can give valuable experience when a person is deciding if a profession is the right one to pursue; interns are often given a ground-level view from which they can observe people who have the job they might hope to have themselves one day.

When a company or organization calls someone an intern, it must follow certain laws and restrictions. An intern must be receiving some substantial career training; an intern cannot be unpaid and completing the same tasks as, or taking the place of, a full-time paid employee. These laws are in place to make sure that employers are dedicated to giving interns the best possible experience without taking advantage of unpaid employees. They are also in place to make sure that employers are not using free help from interns as an excuse not to hire someone.

Introduction

Some young people are able to obtain academic course credit for internship or volunteer opportunities. Talk to your school guidance counselor to see if this is a possibility for you. Even if your school does not directly offer credit, sometimes schools can work in conjunction with local community colleges to help students get academic credit for their experiences that can be applied toward a later college degree. If an internship is completed for academic credit, students might be asked to demonstrate what they've learned through a presentation, a paper, or journal entries chronicling and reflecting on their experience. Academic credit internships may also have more rigorous guidelines to ensure that interns are completing work that is not solely administrative in nature but that also has an academic and professional development component.

Chapter One
RESEARCHING YOUR OUTDOOR INTERESTS

Running, climbing, rowing, swimming, cycling—if you are an athlete, all of these activities probably sound much more appealing than sitting at a desk and working in an office all day. Luckily, interning and volunteering do not have to mean staying still. For young people who want to stay active and still gain new experiences, the key is figuring out what skills you have gained from sports and how they can apply in a setting that is off the court or field.

Brainstorming

To find a fulfilling experience, first think about what you like most about being active. Ask yourself, or talk with another athletic friend about, what makes being active fulfilling to you. Here are some questions to start with:

Researching Your Outdoor Interests

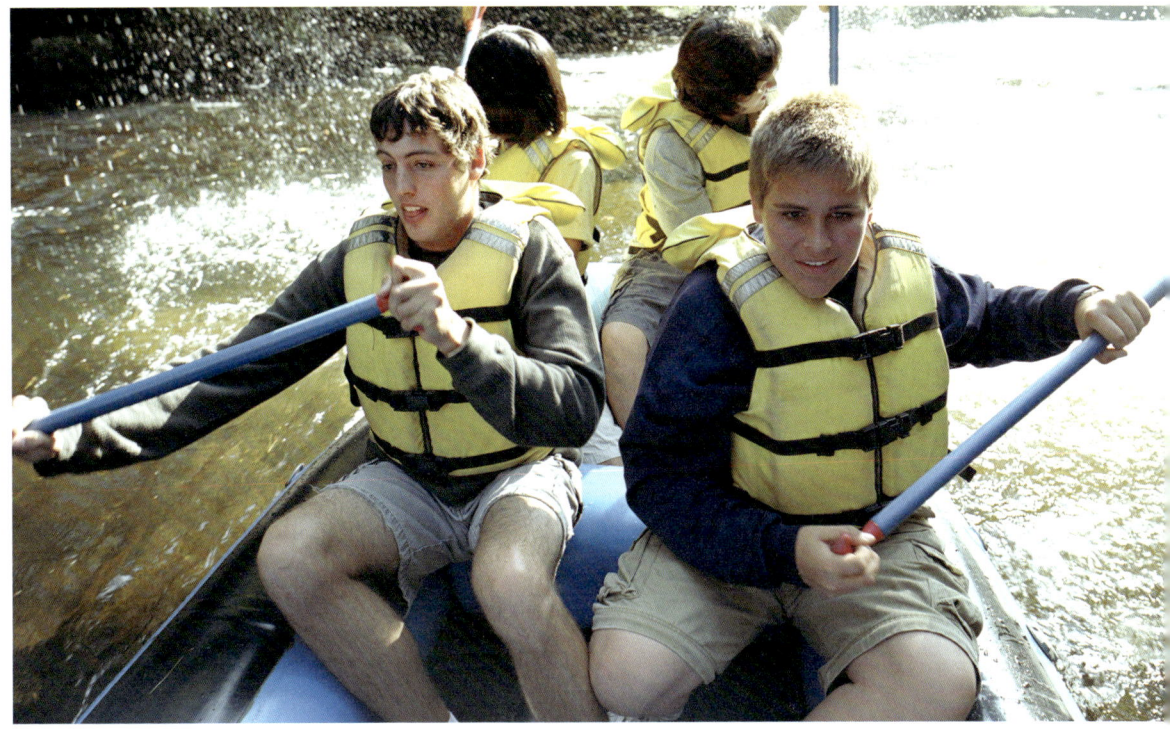

Thinking of your favorite hobbies, such as being on the water, can inspire you in your search for an internship or volunteer opportunity.

- What physical skills does my activity require?
- What mental skills does my activity require?
- What do I like most about my activity?
- Do I prefer team or solo sports?
- What challenges me most about the activities that interest me?

Write down your answers on another piece of paper if it is helpful to you. When you have the answer to these questions, you will

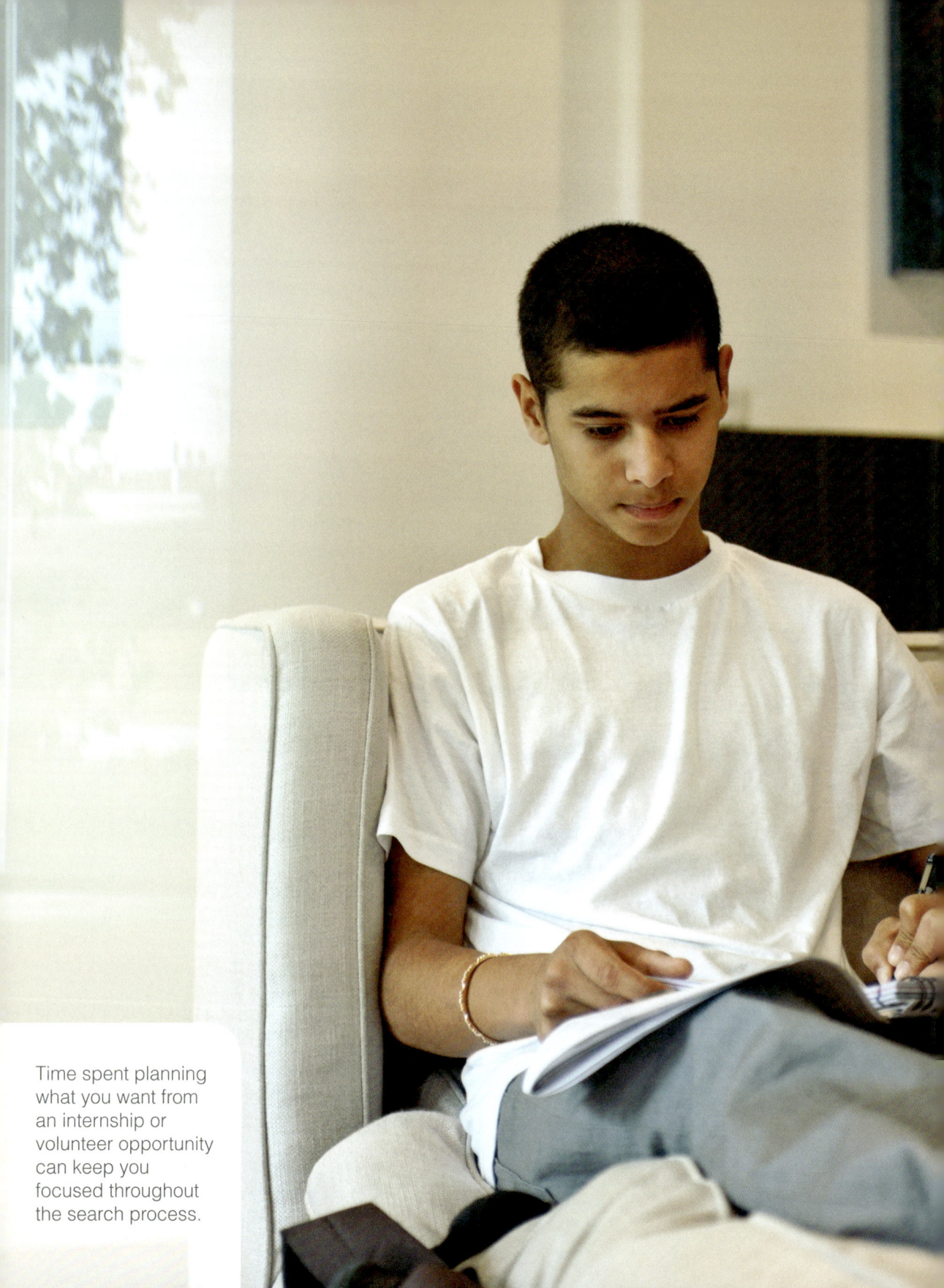

Time spent planning what you want from an internship or volunteer opportunity can keep you focused throughout the search process.

Researching Your Outdoor Interests

be able to ask yourself if the internship or volunteer experiences you are considering will give you the same kind of satisfaction that being active does.

Even an active internship or volunteer opportunity might involve some other types of work, too, so it is helpful to think a little bit about what skills and interests you have outside of your active lifestyle. The best experience for you might be one that combines physical activity with other fields in an unexpected way. Here are some questions to consider by yourself or with a friend:

- What academic subjects do I like most?
- What do I like to do in my free time?
- Do I enjoy working alone or with others? With people my age or with younger or older people?
- Do I prefer to be in charge or to follow someone else's lead?
- Are there particular causes that I feel strongly about?
- Am I an introvert (someone who prefers to keep to himself or herself) or an extrovert (someone who is more outgoing)?
- Am I looking for an experience that gives me new perspective on a familiar topic, or am I looking to branch out into an entirely new field?

Write down or keep in mind your answers to these questions. They will help you focus your search as well as make it clear in your cover letter, résumé, and interview that you are a good fit for a specific experience.

School Resources

Teachers, coaches, guidance counselors, and librarians can all be resources for investigating interests. They have known many students, so they can offer valuable advice about what other young people with similar interests have done in the past. Ask them some of the following questions:

- Have any of their former students pursued an activity-related career?
- What types of skills have their former students mastered that made them attractive candidates for any internship or volunteer opportunities?
- What are ways that one can become more active in the school athletics community?
- What community organizations can they think of that might be a good match for your skills and interests?
- Do they know anyone else whom you might talk to in order to get a new perspective on this subject?

Guidance counselors can give aptitude tests that tell students where their skills lie, and they can help translate these skills and interests to a career field. When you are ready to search, guidance counselors are also often aware of specific opportunities that

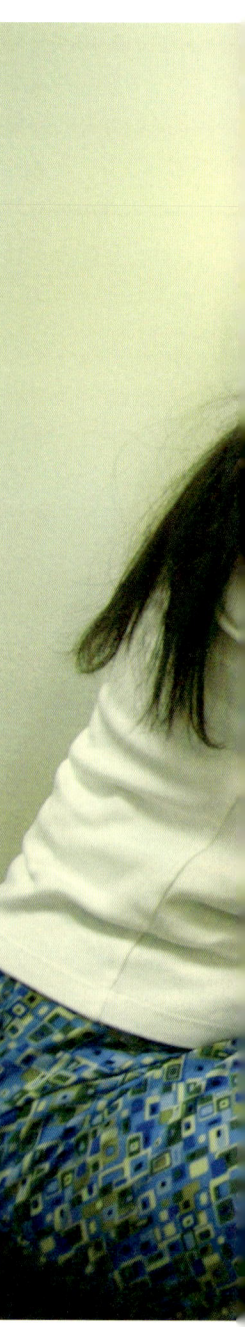

Researching Your Outdoor Interests

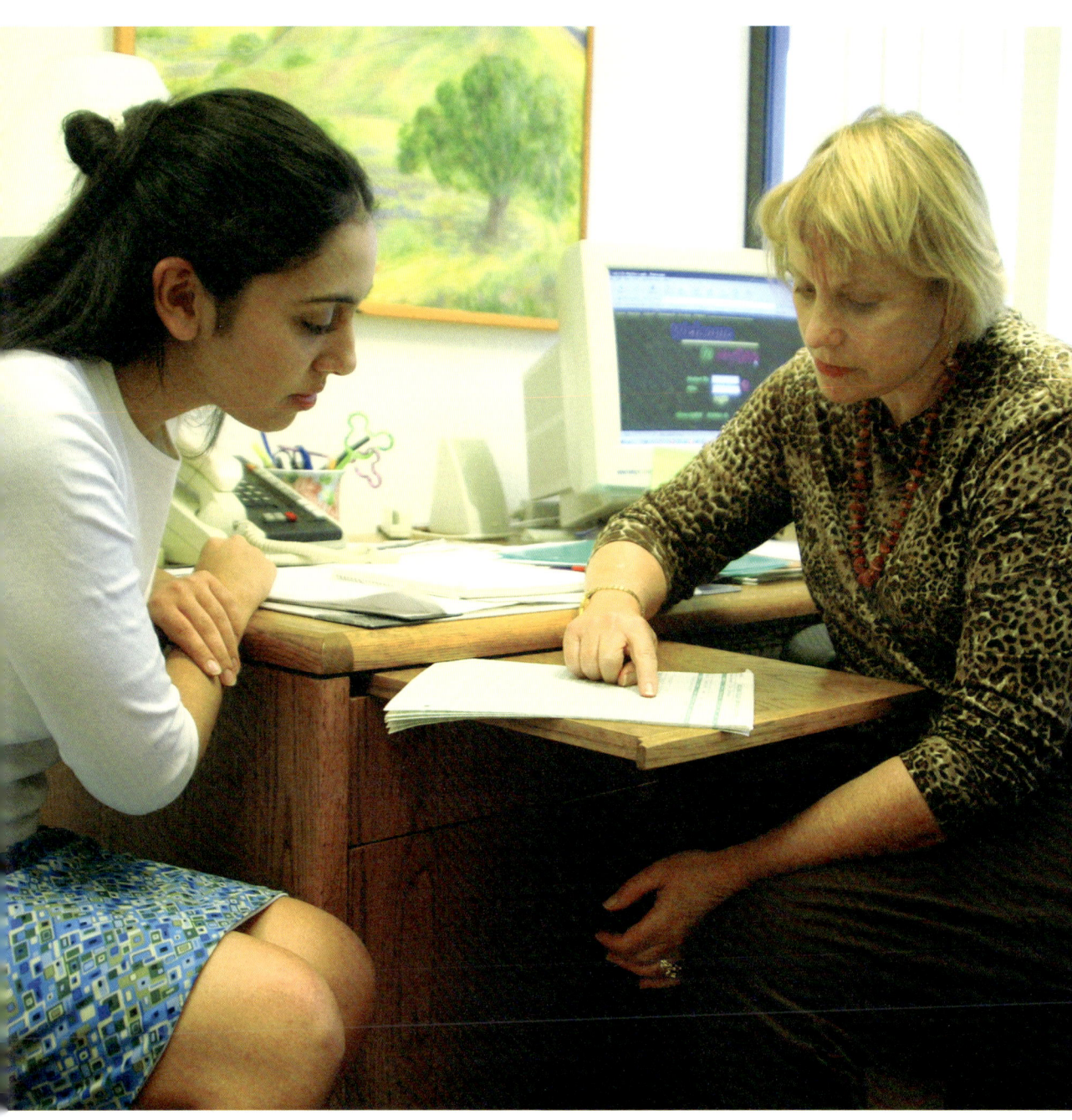

Talking to someone from your school, such as a guidance counselor, can help you figure out how to turn your interests into a career.

are available. If you want or need to receive academic credit for an internship, a guidance counselor can explain the steps to do this and help guide you through any necessary paperwork. Later on, when you are volunteering or interning, a guidance counselor is also a good person to talk to if you have questions or concerns about your experience. Once you have completed the experience, your guidance counselor can also help you figure out how to show off what you have done for future job and college applications.

Librarians are well versed in the art of research. In addition to print resources that they may have in the library, like books and magazines specific to a particular career field, they can also help guide you to general Web sites with career advice and job listings. Your school may have access to subscription-only Web sites that offer information on different career fields. Ask a librarian where the best place to start your information search might be.

The Help of Friends and Family

Your family and friends know you better than anyone else does. Be sure to keep them posted during the investigation process. They might have ideas that are specific just to you on how to apply your interests and skills to a new experience. They can also help you process the information you are finding and keep you from feeling overwhelmed. And of course, their connections to people in your field of interest may help you find the right experience.

Researching Your Outdoor Interests

Books

Your guidance counselor and librarian may have ideas on books that you should check out to help you learn more about your interests, but you might want to look on your own, too. There are several different categories of books that could help you in your research. You can look at general skill assessment books, like the popular *What Color Is Your Parachute*, and books that explain what people in specific fields do.

The resources listed at the end of this book are a good place to start, too. But it is also important to expand your research to books other than those that are just career focused. Check out biographies of your favorite athletes and coaches. Are there organizations they have worked with in the past that interest you? Remember, you are still in the brainstorming stage of your search, so right now, your job is to find ideas that inspire you. Do not be afraid to look off the beaten path.

Internet and Social Media

As with books, you can look at both specific and general Web sites. Your guidance counselor and teacher may have ideas, but look a little further for some less conventional Web sites. From your earlier conversations, you may have names of organizations or people that do something you are interested in. Search for their information, and find out more about what their day-to-day jobs involve.

Do your favorite athletes have Twitter feeds or Facebook pages? If so, what do they tweet about, or what organizations are they fans of? It is a good time to start your own Twitter feed, too. Do

internship & volunteer opportunities for people who love movement

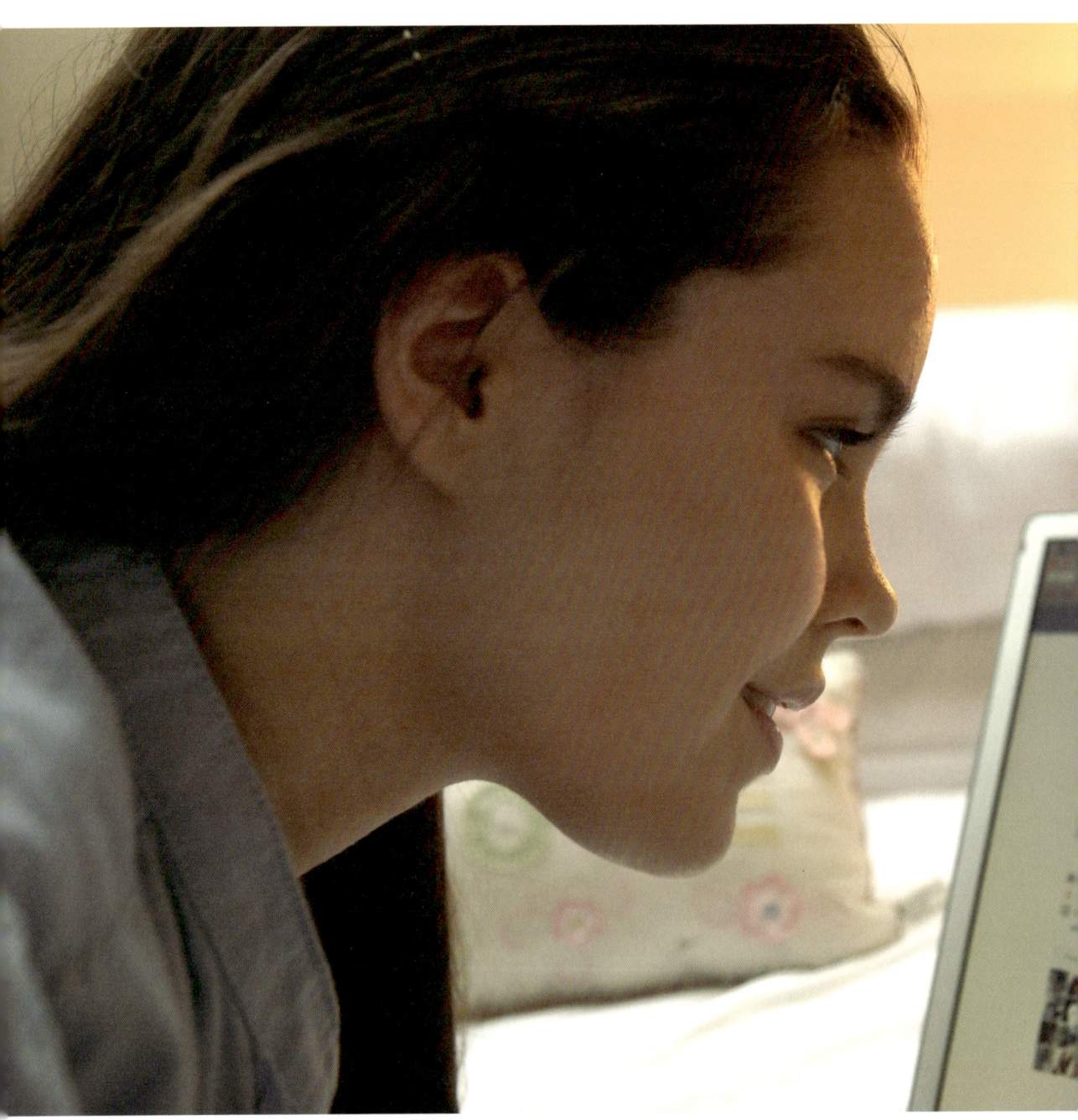

Social networks can be used in creative ways to help sort out career interests and find opportunities through friends and family.

Researching Your Outdoor Interests

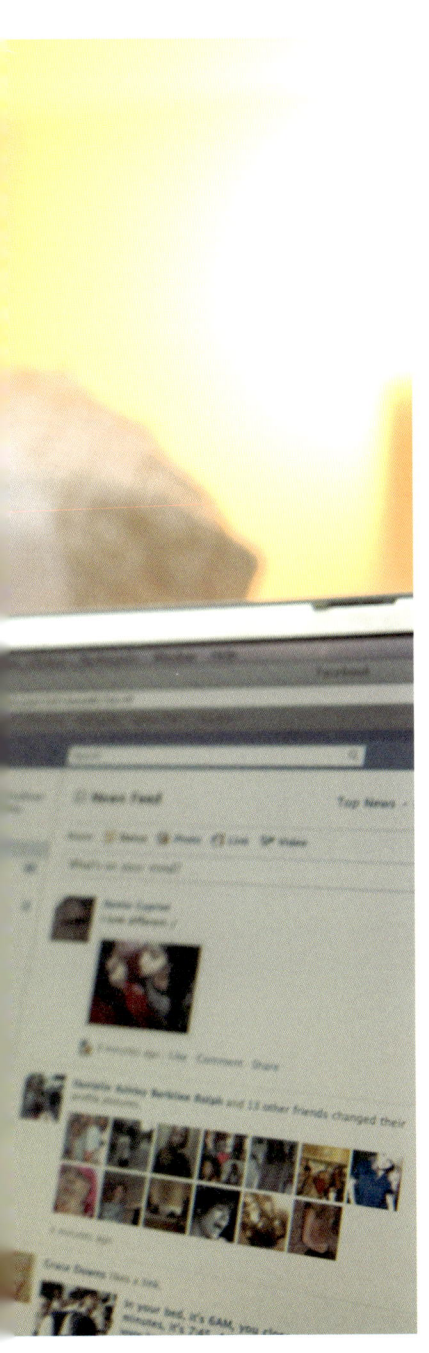

not send out tweets asking people to hire you just yet—for now, focus messages on issues that are relevant to the field in which you would like to work. This will become invaluable when you are ready to search for a specific position; by that time, you will have gained followers who have the same kind of interests as you do and who might be willing to help out.

Blogs are great resources because they offer a less formal look at a person or organization. Try to find one that matches with your interests. If it is an organization that you are interested in, does the tone or personality that is shown through the entries match the type of organization you are looking to work with? If it is an individual person's blog, can you see yourself getting excited about the type of work that he or she is doing?

LinkedIn is a professional networking resource that lists people's work histories. When you link with, or connect to, someone, you can see who else he or she is connected to, too. This is helpful as you are researching a field in several ways. First, by viewing people's work history, you can learn how they reached their position and what other jobs they have held in the past. This might give you new ideas for experiences you might like to have. Second, as you learn who your acquaintances know, you may find that you are closely connected to a person at an organization that you are interested in working with or finding out more about.

Informational Interviews

Now that you have talked to many of your acquaintances, you may have found that you are connected to someone who works in a field that interests you. While you are still brainstorming, the next step is to reach out to that person to request an informational interview. Ask your connection to help facilitate this by passing on a polite e-mail asking for a quick ten- or fifteen-minute conversation. Right now, you are not asking about open positions; you are looking to learn more about the field and how to make yourself an appealing candidate for future positions. If you do not have a personal connection, use the Internet, including searching on Facebook, Twitter, and LinkedIn, to contact someone, explaining your interest and asking for a quick conversation. Many people like to talk about what they do, and since you are making it clear that you are looking for career information and not asking to be hired for a specific job, it takes away the pressure of a conversation. Of course, if a volunteer or internship position opens up later on, the informational interview helps you stand out as a candidate for your interest.

Before going into an informational interview, review everything you know about the field, and research the organization or company. Make a list of the questions you would like to ask—it is helpful if you order them from most important to least, in case you run out of time. Offer to send these questions to the person ahead of time

Researching Your Outdoor Interests

so that he or she has time to think about the answers. Some good places to start are: What do you like about your job? What is the most challenging part of your position? What type of education and experience prepared you for this career field? Are there other similar careers that you considered? What does your organization look for in hiring an intern or volunteer? What are some of the typical tasks of interns or volunteers at your organization? Be sure to follow up your meeting with a thank-you note for the person's time.

If you cannot meet with someone face to face—either because of the distance or because the person does not have time—e-mail can serve as a valuable tool for this conversation as well.

Reflect on what you learn about different fields and your own interests as you go through this information-gathering process. Taking the time at the beginning to learn about what you want will pay off later when you are considering if a specific experience is the right one for you.

Chapter Two

FINDING OPPORTUNITIES

Now it is time to find (and get hired for!) a volunteer or internship opportunity that matches your needs. From your previous exploration, you probably have a good idea of the type of work that you would like to do—maybe you have even spoken with someone who works with a company or organization you like. Even if your research has given you only a general idea, do not worry. Wanting to learn more about a field is a good reason to volunteer or intern, and it is OK—and even helpful—if after a few weeks or months in your position you realize that you do not want to make a career out of it.

Depending on the position and company, the application process may be more or less complicated. Some organizations are happy to take any volunteers who offer, and others may have a limited number of spots or have specific age or education requirements, which means they will have a more extensive process. Be sure to check that you fit the requirements before you apply; it will save

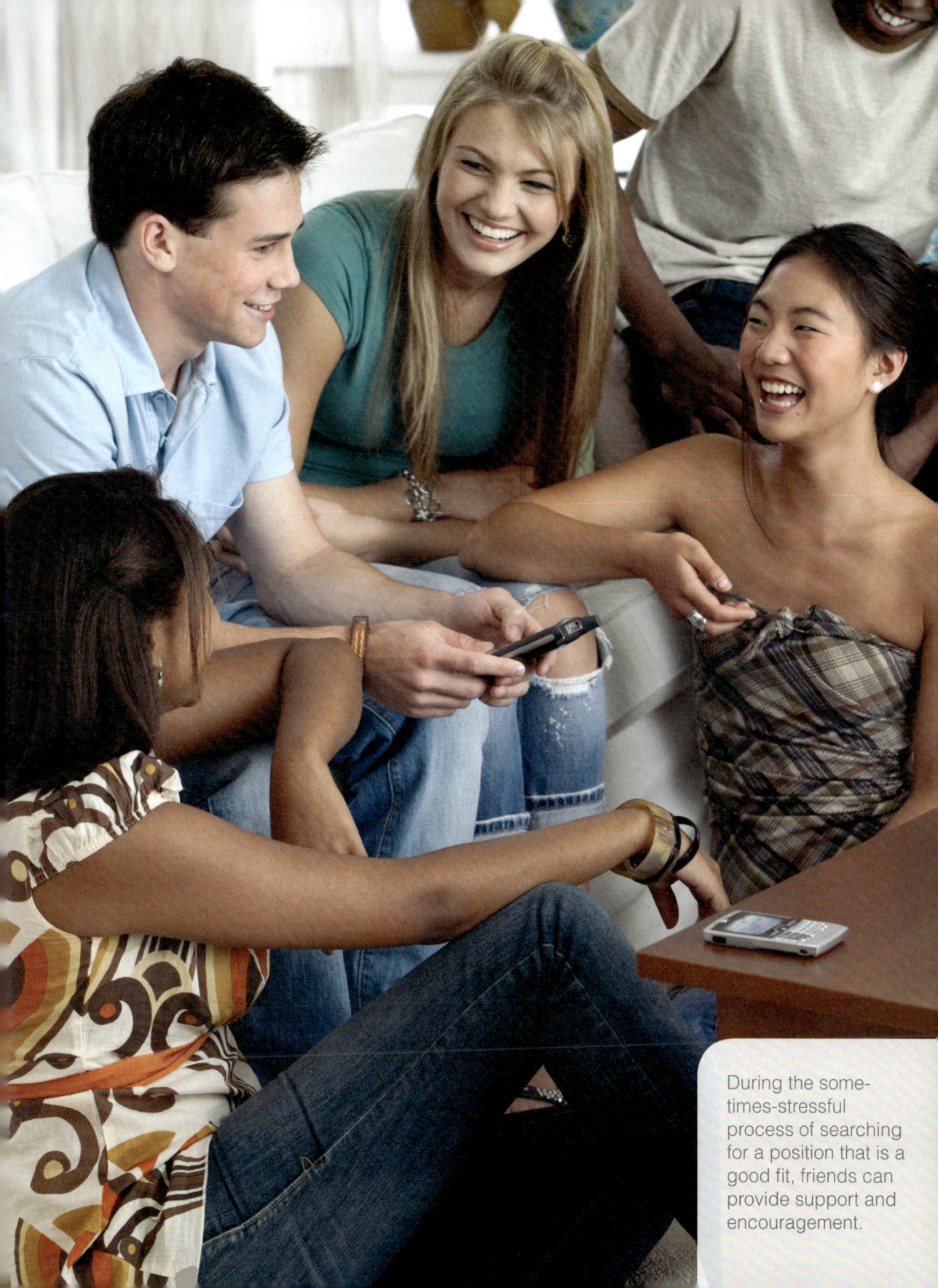

During the sometimes-stressful process of searching for a position that is a good fit, friends can provide support and encouragement.

you time in the long run. If an internship or volunteer opportunity is not a good fit for you right now but might work in the future, be sure to keep a note of it for the next time that you are searching.

Personal Connections

As with the information-gathering process, your family and friends will again be a great source for helping you find a specific position. Now that you know more about what you are interested in, make sure you spread the word. Maybe your little sister's T-ball team is looking for a volunteer coach, or your best friend's aunt is a personal trainer looking for an intern to help out. Your family and friends will not know to mention you if you do not tell them you are looking, so get the word out.

Check back in with teachers, coaches, and guidance counselors, too. Sometimes organizations looking for athletic young people to help out will go straight to these people and ask for recommendations. If you remind them that you are looking for this type of opportunity, you will be the first person they think of.

Now is also the time to check back in with people you had informational interviews with. A polite e-mail can remind them of your interest. To show them that you valued their input, mention a couple of details from your conversation. Try saying something like this:

Dear Ms. Lorenzo,

Thank you again for meeting with me last month. Since we spoke, I've been thinking more about teaching yoga, especially about your comments regarding mixing discipline with the knowledge of each student's abilities. I'm very interested in this field and am currently looking for an internship or volunteer opportunity to learn more. If you hear of any openings or have any recommendations for me, would you please let me know?

*Sincerely,
Jonathan*

Searching Online

Online searching is a big part of modern-day job hunting. There are some major national Web sites, such as Monster, and some job sites that are specialized to your location, such as Craigslist or your local newspaper's online want ads. Opportunities listed on these larger Web sites can sometimes be competitive; since the Web sites are the first thing many people think of when searching, there may be more applicants. If there are particular organizations that you are interested in, you should check the listings on their individual Web sites.

Social networking offers other unconventional opportunities for online job searching, too. If you have already established a presence on Twitter, it is a good time to send out a tweet saying that you are looking to intern or volunteer and asking anyone who can help to send you a message. Use this sparingly; you still want your Twitter feed to focus on your subject matter to show your expertise instead of being taken over by your job search—but do not be afraid to send a couple of messages out each week. You never know who is reading you.

internship & volunteer opportunities for people who love movement

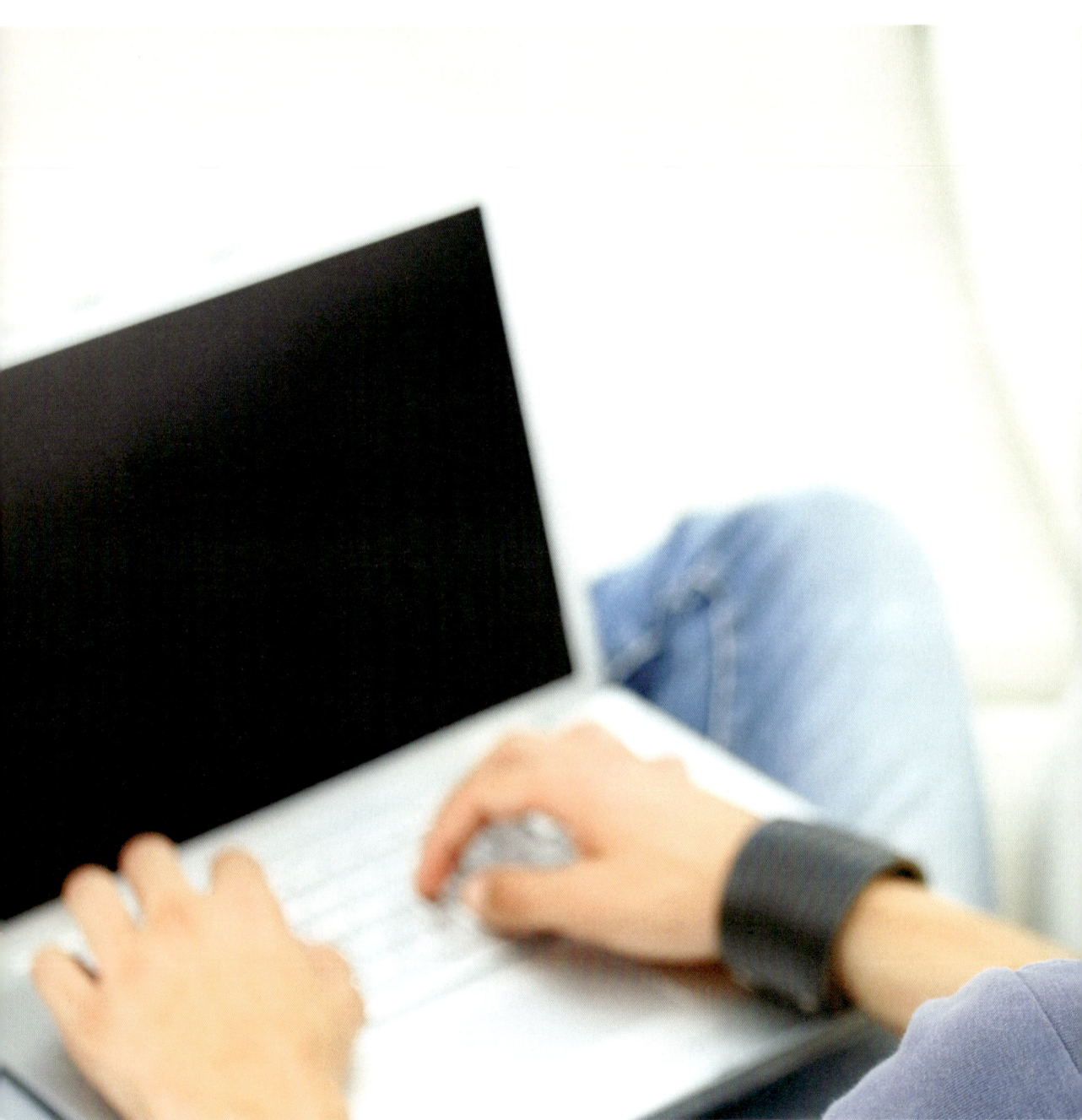

The first step in finding the right opportunity for you is searching online.

> **Finding Opportunities**

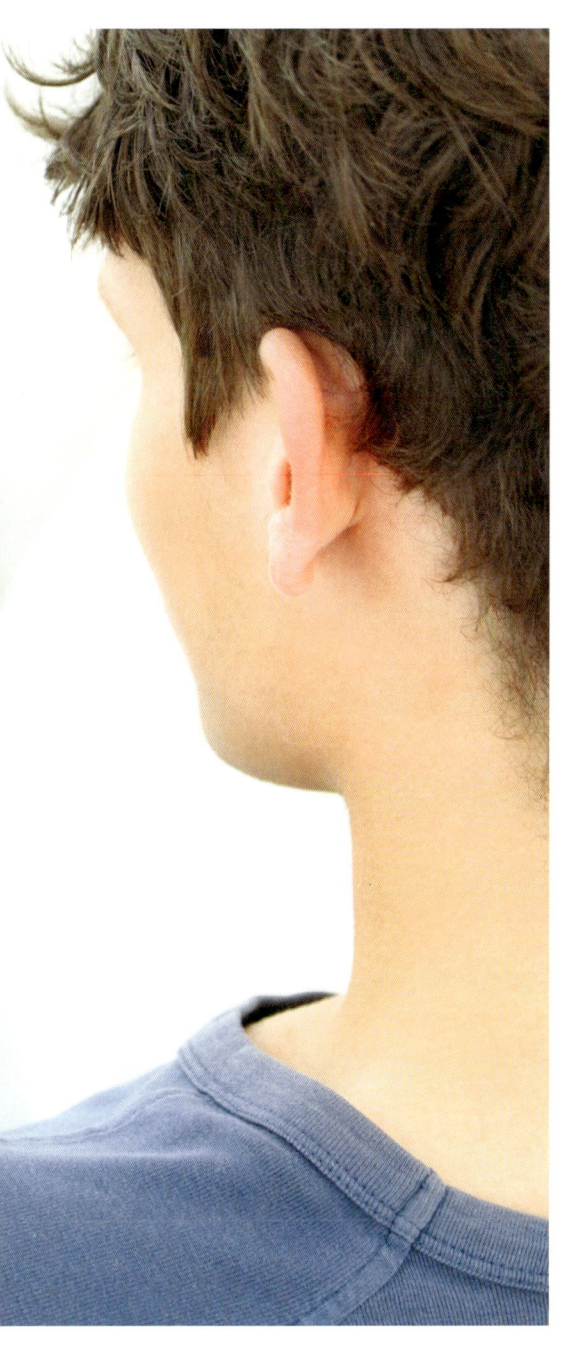

If you are on LinkedIn, update your profile to reflect your interest and any experience you might have in the field, and make sure that you have reached out to all of your connections who might be able to help. If you are applying for a specific position with a company or organization, check to see if you have any connections who work there.

On Facebook, write a status update to let your friends know the type of position you are looking for and become fans of organizations and companies that interest you. And make sure that all of your social networking Web sites are either set to private or do not have any information, comments, or photographs that could offend a prospective employer.

Local Resources

You have asked your friends and family for ideas, and you have searched online, but sometimes it is a neighbor who has just the

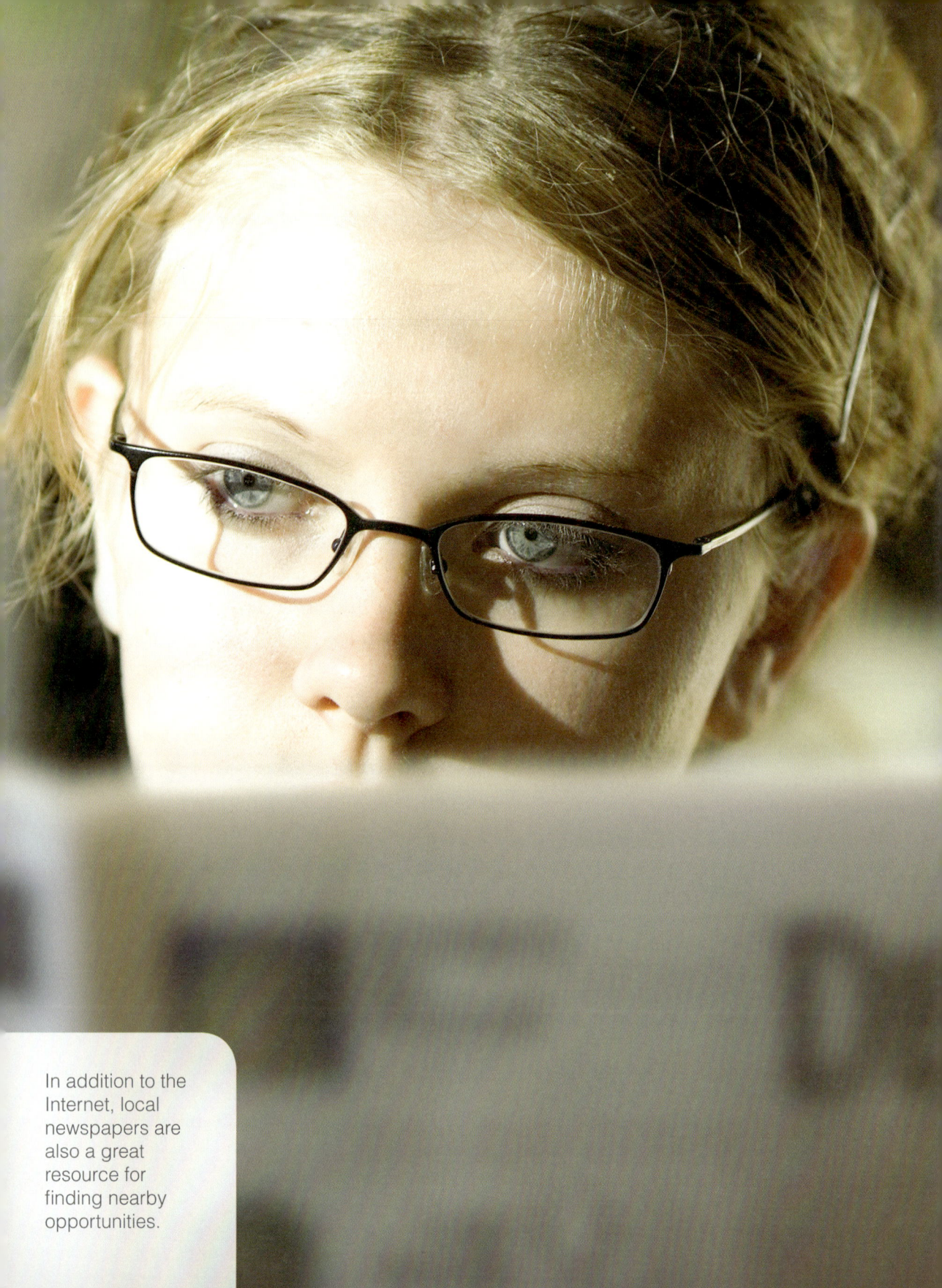

In addition to the Internet, local newspapers are also a great resource for finding nearby opportunities.

Finding Opportunities

opportunity for you. Keep your eye out for listings in local newspapers and newsletters. Reach out to local community centers, cafes, and libraries and ask if you can put flyers up explaining the kind of position that you are looking for. If you are looking to volunteer as a coach, ask schools, community centers, and established local teams if they need anyone. And do not forget about the phone book, either—it may seem old-fashioned, but sometimes flipping through will remind you of local organizations or companies that would be perfect fits.

Sometimes these local organizations might not have an internship or volunteer program set up but are interested in your help. If that is the case, you can work with them to create a new opportunity. Be ready to tell them how you are looking to help and what types of skills you have to offer. Whether this opportunity becomes a formal program or is an informal agreement, you are still getting the same valuable experience.

Cover Letters

For some positions, you will need to write a cover letter. A cover letter is a brief introduction to you and your past experience, and it explains why you are interested in or a good fit for a particular job. Your résumé will give you the opportunity to list specific information about your previous positions or experiences. The cover letter is the place to use examples to make it clear why this job is right for you. A résumé might include a volunteer coaching position and list the number of games won. A cover letter might say what you learned from your experience coaching—for example, how to encourage a group of young beginner players as well as how to analyze and enact the best defensive strategies on the soccer field.

Making Résumés Work for You

Did you know that there are different ways you can format a résumé? Depending on how much experience you have, and the position you are applying for, you can choose to focus on relevant skills, relevant work, or relevant education.

Some opportunities might require you to submit a résumé summarizing your experience. Do not worry; if the company or organization is open to young interns or volunteers, then they do not expect you to have tons of experience—and you probably have more to offer than you realize. A résumé can include after-school jobs and previous volunteer or internship experiences, but it can also include extracurricular activities, like sports teams and clubs, and relevant academic experiences. Think back to the brainstorming you did while you were identifying what skills you have to offer. If you are a science whiz, then state your anatomy knowledge on that résumé that you are sending in to the personal trainer.

In general, résumés can include any mix of:

- Skills—list any general skills that are relevant to the particular position, such as strong communication skills or experience with younger children.

Finding Opportunities

- Education—you can expand this section to mention relevant classes and research projects.
- Experience—include athletic experiences as well as past volunteer or internship positions.
- Extracurricular activities—include clubs, positions held, and activities participated in.
- Awards—do not forget to mention your athletic achievements here, too.

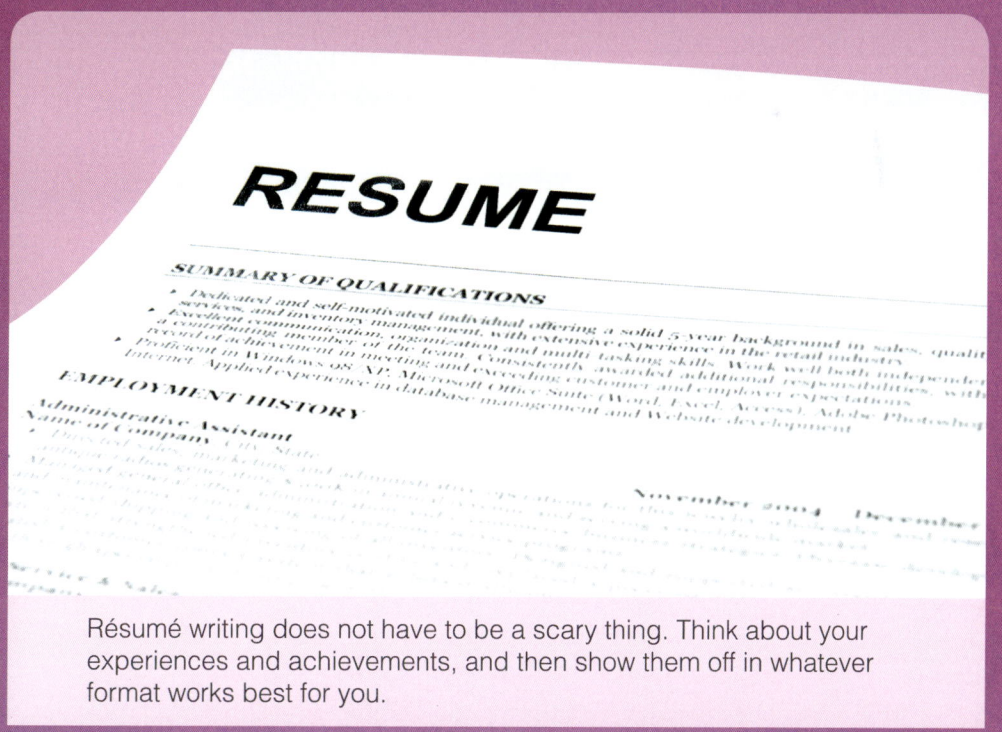

Résumé writing does not have to be a scary thing. Think about your experiences and achievements, and then show them off in whatever format works best for you.

internship & volunteer opportunities for people who love movement

Acing the Interview

Finally, you have been called in for an interview! You have done a lot of research by now, so you should know what the general field does, and you probably know a bit about what the organization or company does, too. Brush up on the specifics of the company or organization before you go in for your interview and think of a few questions you have about the position.

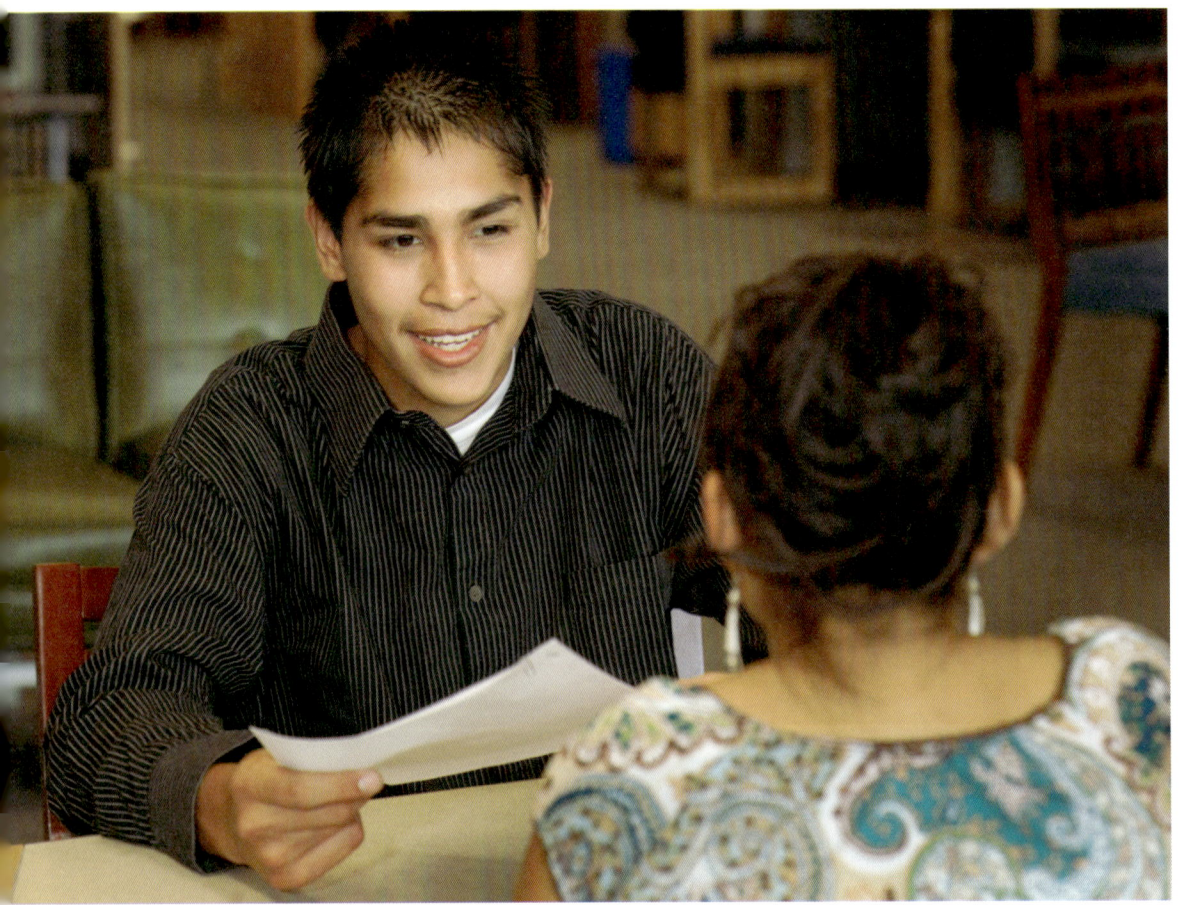

Asking questions in interviews is a way to learn more about the day-to-day life at a company or organization.

Finding Opportunities

    These questions might be similar to ones that you would ask at an informational interview, but this time, they should all be focused on the specific position. Do you know what you would be doing on a day-to-day basis? Who would you go to if you need help? How long will the experience last? On the day of the interview, wear a nice outfit, arrive on time, and relax! It is not just about the organization asking questions of you—it is a time for you to learn if the position is right for you, too. Follow up the interview with a thank-you note. If they offer you a position, accept or decline promptly and politely. Be sure to keep everyone who helped you along the way posted on your progress.

Chapter Three

COACHING

For many active young people looking to volunteer or intern in an area related to movement, coaching is the first logical choice, and the one most closely linked to their own interests. Athletes spend years building their skills in a sport, so they are true experts on the subject. As a career choice, it offers players the opportunity to stay in the game even after their playing years are over. As an interning or volunteering choice, it offers young people the opportunity to sharpen observations about the game and help teach others who may just be starting to learn the sport.

A coach's job varies depending on how serious the athlete or team he or she coaches is. For coaches that teach kids who are just learning a sport, the job focuses on teaching good sportsmanship, the importance of teamwork, and how to play without getting hurt or hurting someone

Coaching

else. As kids get older, coaches focus more on relaying skills and planning strategies specific to defeating other teams. Coaches analyze the game, watching what players are doing correctly and advising on places that need improvement. When athletes reach the high school level, coaches take on the added responsibility of helping their college-bound athletes train and compete

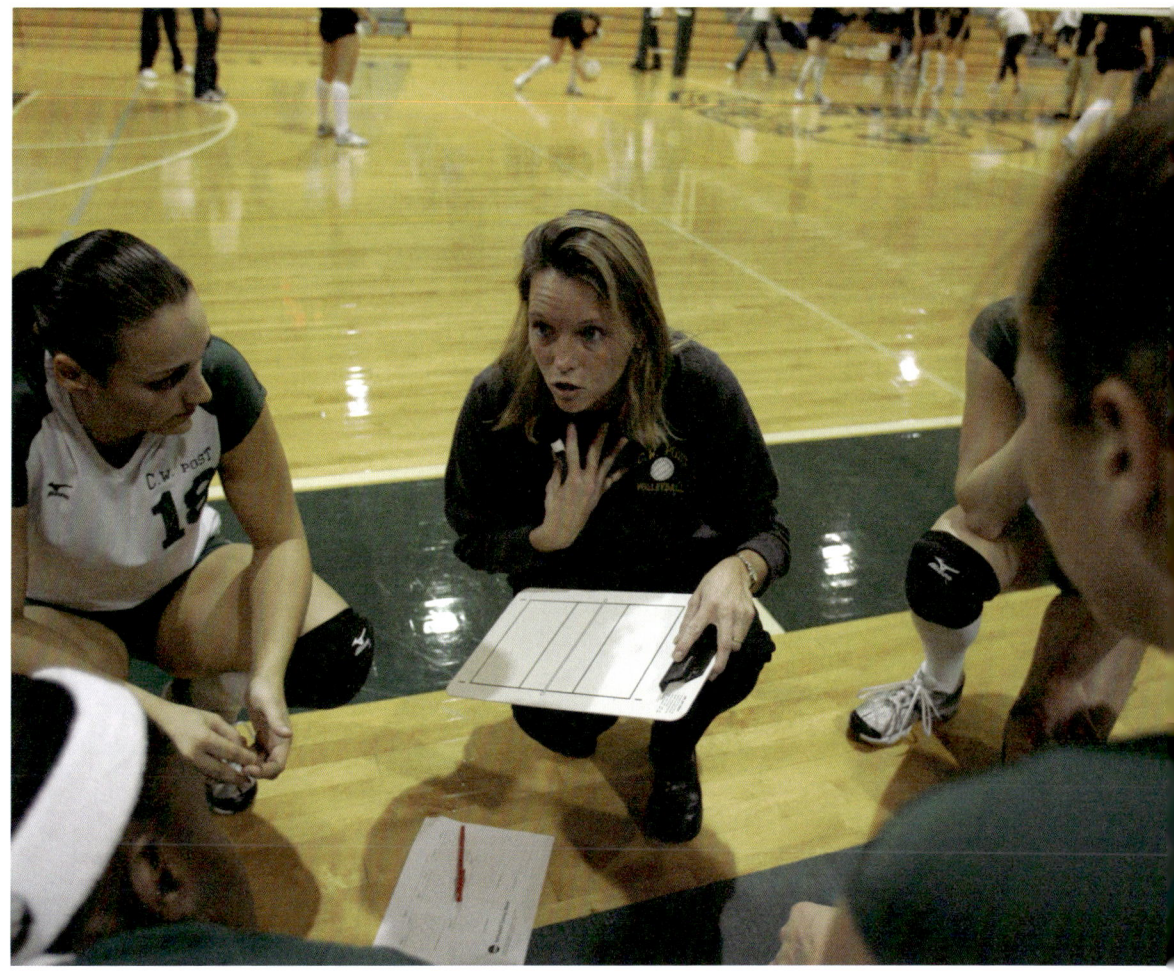

Careers in coaching often start with internships as a coach's assistant, which is a great way to learn the ropes.

for scholarships. At a college and professional level, coaches are often held accountable for their teams' performances, and their jobs can depend on it. Their job is to create a team that takes into account each player's strengths and weaknesses—and uses this knowledge to win.

Team sports often involve a close-knit group of people, and coaches can be at the helm of this, encouraging group bonding and emphasizing to student athletes the importance of excelling in the classroom as well. This means that coaches can take on the role of mentor both in the sport and in life in general.

Legendary Coaches

At some colleges, coaches are closely linked to school spirit and identity. Penn State University's longtime coach, Joe Paterno, was one of the most well-known and beloved coaches in college football history, and he holds the record for coaching winning games in NCAA Division I. When he was fired after a sex abuse scandal broke involving an assistant coach in 2011, shocked students and alumni took to the streets of State College, Pennsylvania, to protest, saying that without him the school didn't have an identity. Paterno died a few months later.

Coaching

Some coaches are hired directly by schools. Other coaches are hired by community centers. Although many coaches work with children, intramural sports for adults is also growing in popularity. Some senior citizen centers also offer sports for their residents. Some businesses even offer recreational sports teams for their employees. All of these groups need skilled and dedicated players who are willing to teach the sport.

Coaching offers the opportunity to work in any sport you can find or create a team for. T-ball, baseball, softball, soccer, basketball, and volleyball are some of the most popular team sports.

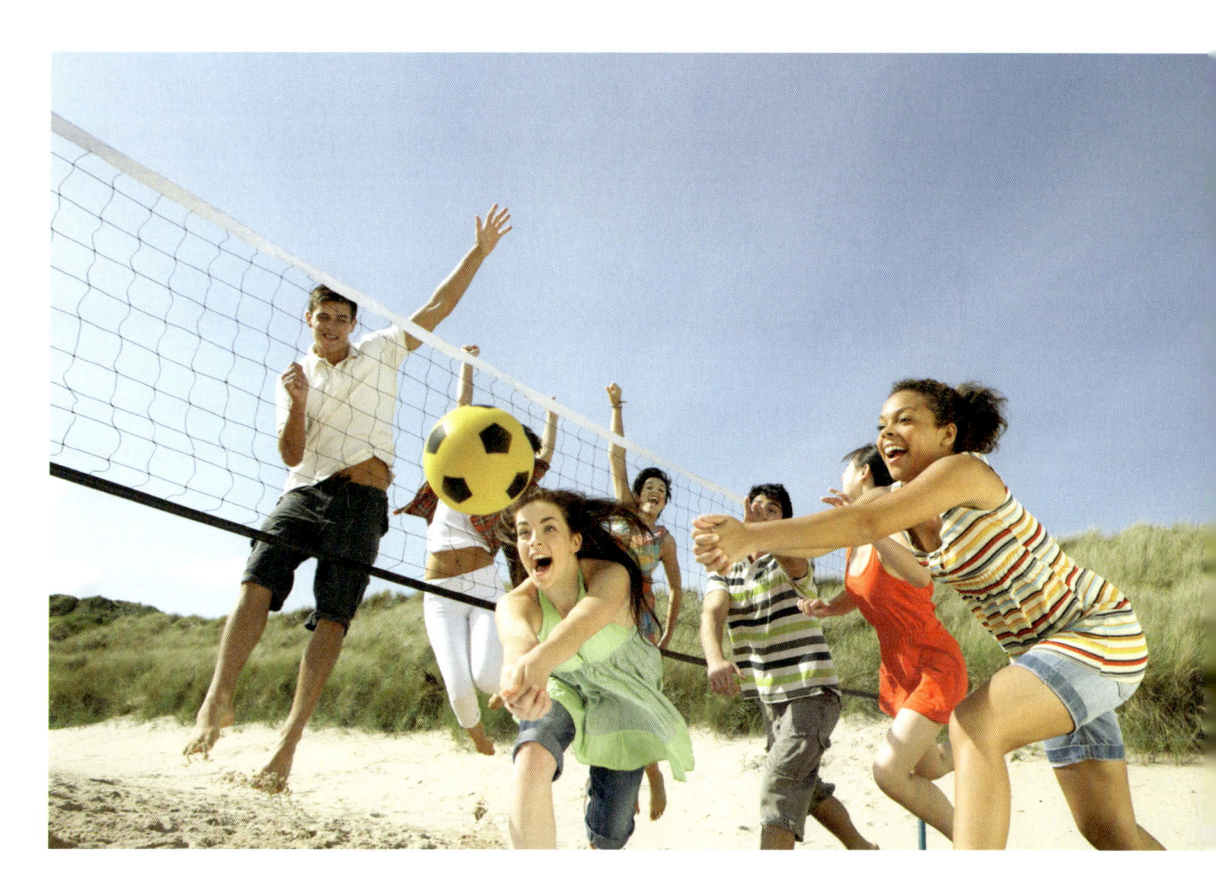

Coaches work with teams of varying skill levels, from people who want to become professionals to those who are looking for a fun weekend activity.

internship & volunteer opportunities for people who love movement

You might also help coach swimming, tennis, track and field, gymnastics, or golf.

To be a successful coach, you should be dedicated to the sport you are coaching, you should be able to explain simply and demonstrate basic and advanced moves, and you should enjoy teaching others both the rules and the love of the game.

What Interning or Volunteering Might Mean

Some less formal community sports groups might allow a young athlete to coach his or her own team. Other groups might ask a young person to serve as an assistant coach. Volunteers or interns can expect to help run practices, demonstrate specific skills, coordinate drills, and work one-on-one to help individuals master particular moves. Volunteers can also expect to help keep team spirit up, arguments down, and demonstrate good sportsmanship, especially if they are working with younger children.

Where to Look

Start by asking coaches directly if they need help or if they know another team that does. Approach community centers and ask if they have sports programs. If they do not have a sports program, ask if they are interested in starting one. Your or your friends' younger siblings may play on teams that could use an extra hand.

Chapter Four

TEACHING

For athletics that are not team-based, people often learn or practice by taking classes led by instructors. Active young people who have spent years rehearsing dance pirouettes, perfecting downward facing dog yoga positions, and striving toward their black belts might find that helping out with a class is the right intern or volunteer opportunity for them.

Yoga

In recent years, yoga's popularity has soared. It is now offered to everyone from young people to senior citizens. And the sport has developed in different directions as well—some forms of yoga, such as ashtanga, are physically strenuous and provide active workouts. Other types, such as ananda, focus more on breathing and meditation. There is even a type of yoga,

internship & volunteer opportunities for people who love movement

Is Yoga for Everyone?

Because of yoga's recent popularity, injuries have also increased in the sport. An article in the *New York Times Magazine* suggested that this might be because the sport has become more of a competition than it has been in the past, with participants who are not used to physical activity striving to match their classmates' poses and stretching themselves farther than their bodies can handle. For this reason, it is important that anyone teaching yoga pay attention to correct body alignment and emphasizes that students should be aware of their own body's pain and limits.

called bikram, where participants pose, stretch, and move in a room heated to at least 95 degrees Fahrenheit (35 degrees Celsius).

Since there are so many types of yoga, it is important to make sure that an organization that you intern or volunteer with matches your style and expertise. The classes are different paces and have different purposes. Some are primarily exercise, but others have a spiritual and meditative focus.

An intern or volunteer at a yoga studio may be called on to demonstrate the proper way to perform poses. They might also

Teaching

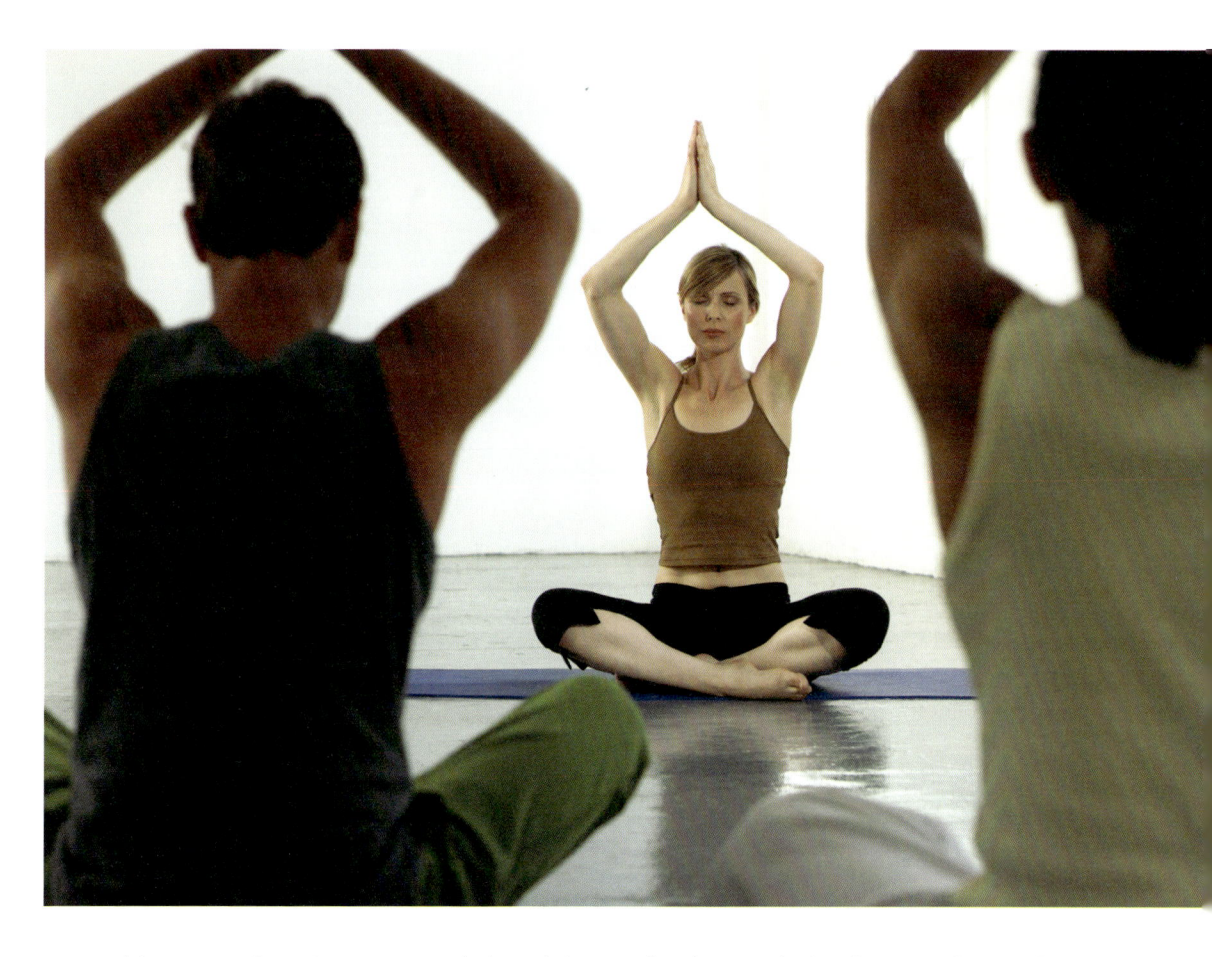

Many people enjoy yoga, and since it is growing in popularity, there are increasing volunteer and internship opportunities with seasoned instructors.

help gently correct students while not forcing someone beyond his or her abilities. And because people are attracted to yoga for different reasons, interns or volunteers might find themselves helping students determine which type of yoga is right for their own needs.

Pilates

Though it has not quite reached the same level of familiarity as yoga, Pilates is another form of exercise that has gained popularity in recent years. It was established by Joseph Pilates in the early 1900s and involves a series of exercises that work to strengthen the body's core, or abdominal and back muscles, while maintaining proper breathing techniques. The sport's focus is on performing the movements correctly rather than repetition, so an intern or volunteer should be quite familiar with the technique before helping out.

As with yoga, an intern or volunteer may model movements and correct students. Since Pilates exercises can be intensified depending on a class's skill level, an intern or volunteer could also be helpful to a teacher in observing and assessing when students are prepared for a more advanced workout.

Dance

Dance is filled with rich variance—jazz, ballet, modern, hip-hop, and tap

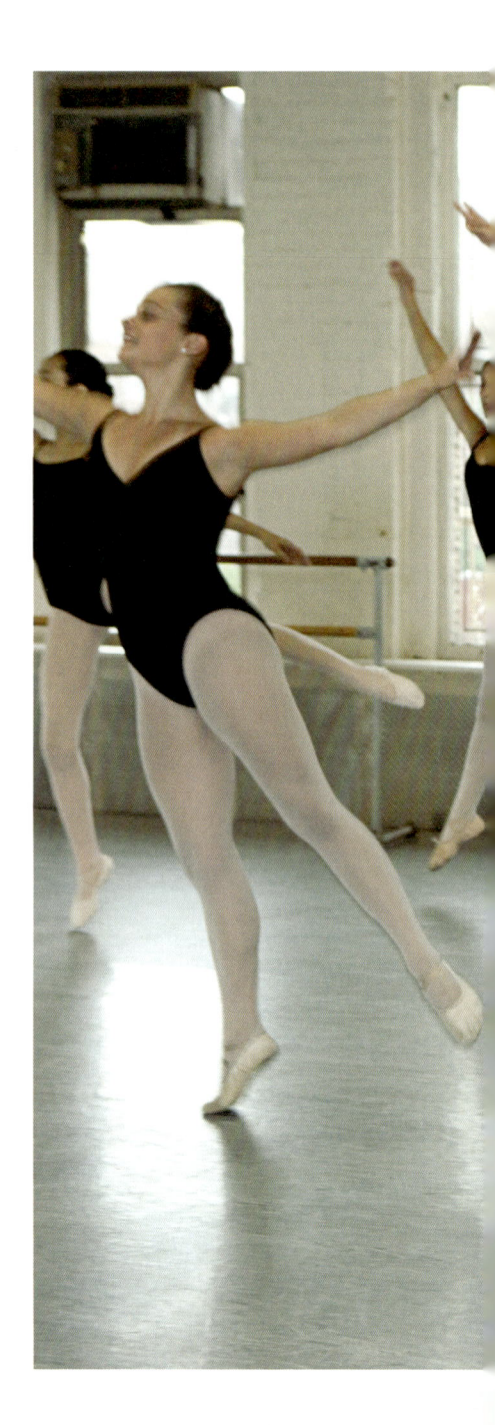

Teaching

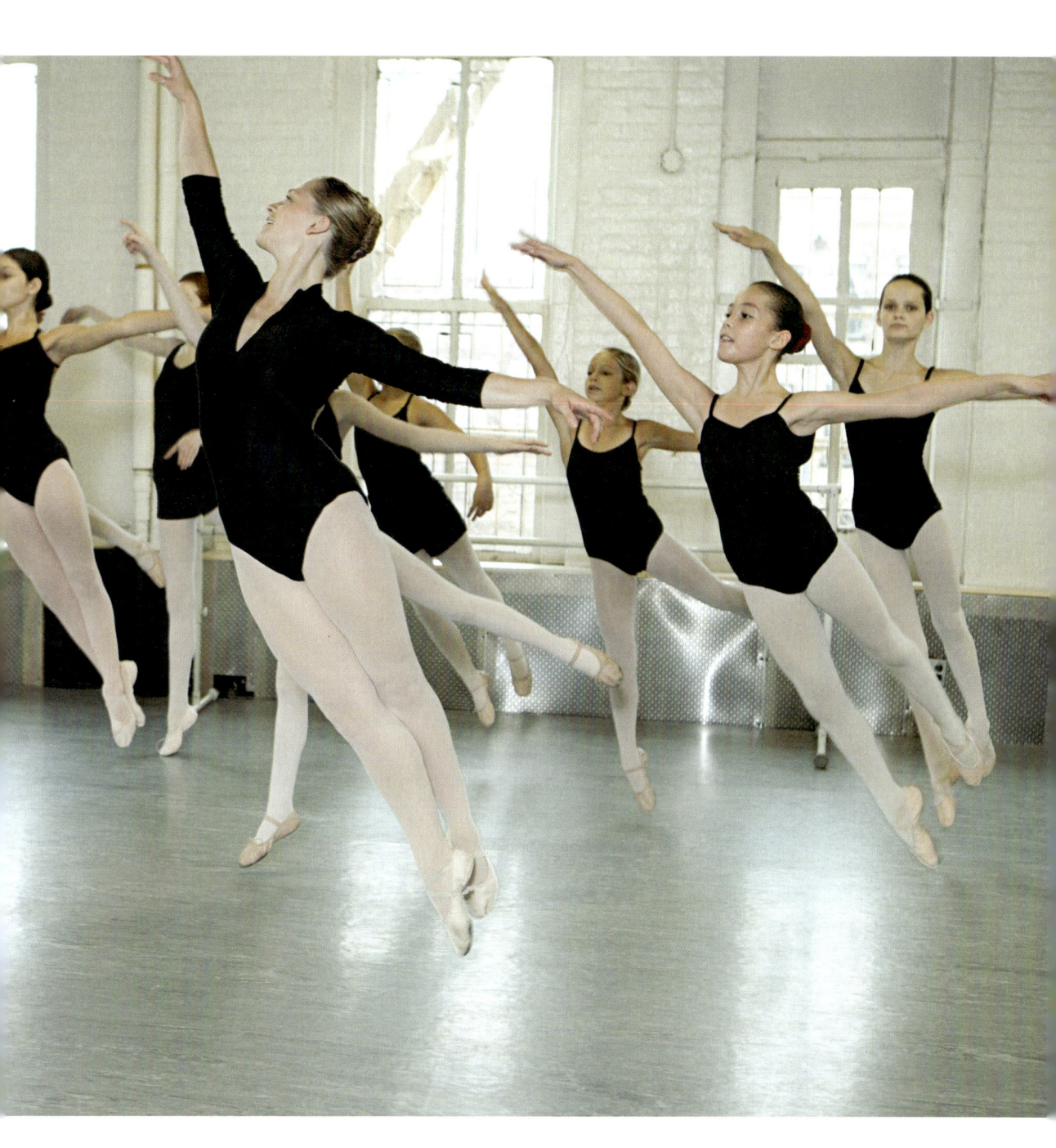

Dance requires discipline, athletic ability, and creativity, so someone with all of these skills has the potential to excel in a volunteer or intern position.

are some of the most popular. Many dancers have participated in the sport for years, so they are familiar with the blend of creativity and discipline required both to participate in a class and to help teach one.

A volunteer or intern at a dance class for amateur or younger dancers will model poses and correct students, as well as instill a love of the sport. Some interns or volunteers for amateur dancers might also be called on to find music and help choreograph, or plan the steps to, a dance. For more advanced dancers, volunteers or interns would not do as much modeling or correction, but they might observe the class and let the instructor know where in the choreography dancers struggled or needed additional instruction. A volunteer or intern might also help with preparing for a performance by assisting with costumes or sets.

Martial Arts

Martial arts encompass many variations: karate, tae kwon do, jujitsu, and kickboxing are some of the most familiar ones in America, though there are countless other varieties all around the world. Martial arts are sports that involve physical combat between people. Similar to yoga, martial arts practices do historically have a spiritual and meditative component to them. Today, people practice for a variety of reasons, including self-defense as well as learning confidence and discipline. Before interning or volunteering with a martial arts class, it is helpful to know if the instructor has a similar outlook on the sport as you do: how spiritual the practice is, for example, and when it is OK to use what is taught in class.

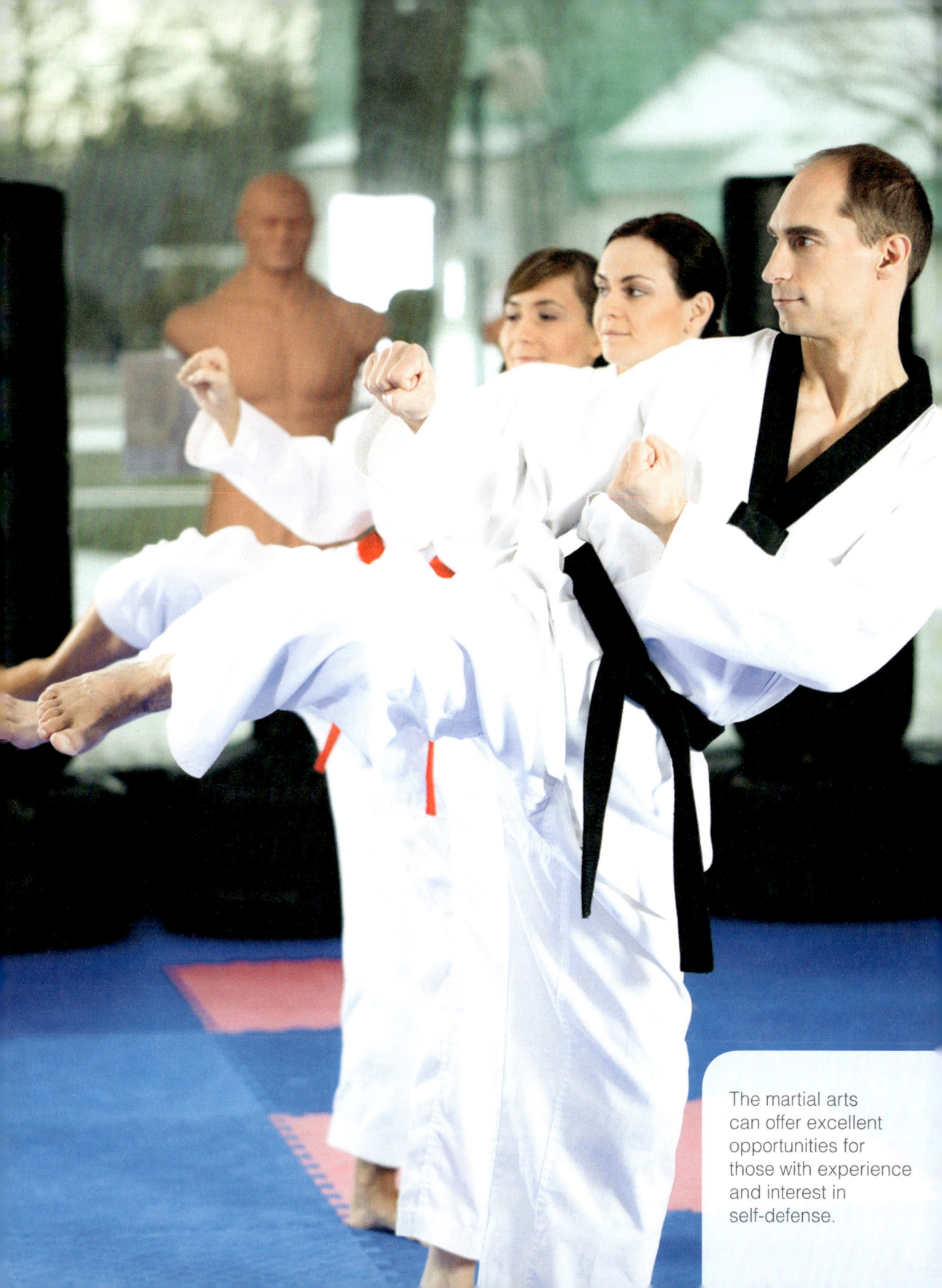

The martial arts can offer excellent opportunities for those with experience and interest in self-defense.

internship & volunteer opportunities for people who love movement

Interns or volunteers in a martial arts class may join with the teacher to demonstrate particular moves. They may also pair up with students to practice as necessary and watch to make sure that no student accidentally harms another. Because this is a sport that does involve a form of fighting, volunteers and interns may also be called on to act as role models, showing and discussing when it is OK to use the sport out of the classroom.

Where to Look

Local gyms and community centers offer both onetime and ongoing classes for a variety of sports at all age and ability levels. Ask an instructor or director for advice on whom to talk to about helping out. Look in the phone book or search online to find local yoga, Pilates, dance, and martial arts studios.

Chapter Five

WORKING WITH INDIVIDUALS

Coaching a team and teaching a class can be fulfilling because of the opportunity to work with so many people at once. But for those who prefer to work more intensively one-on-one with people, there are plenty of active ways to do that, too.

Personal Trainer

When people have a particular fitness goal they wish to meet, they sometimes hire personal trainers. Personal trainers work with individuals to assess their past athletic experiences, their nutritional habits, any type of injury, their current abilities, and their goals for the future. This specific knowledge allows personal trainers to create exercise programs designed to meet the goal. Personal trainers often observe and assist with workouts as well, providing feedback on what a person is doing well and where improvements are needed. Personal trainers can

Personal trainers help individuals create and meet their own physical fitness goals and feel better about themselves overall.

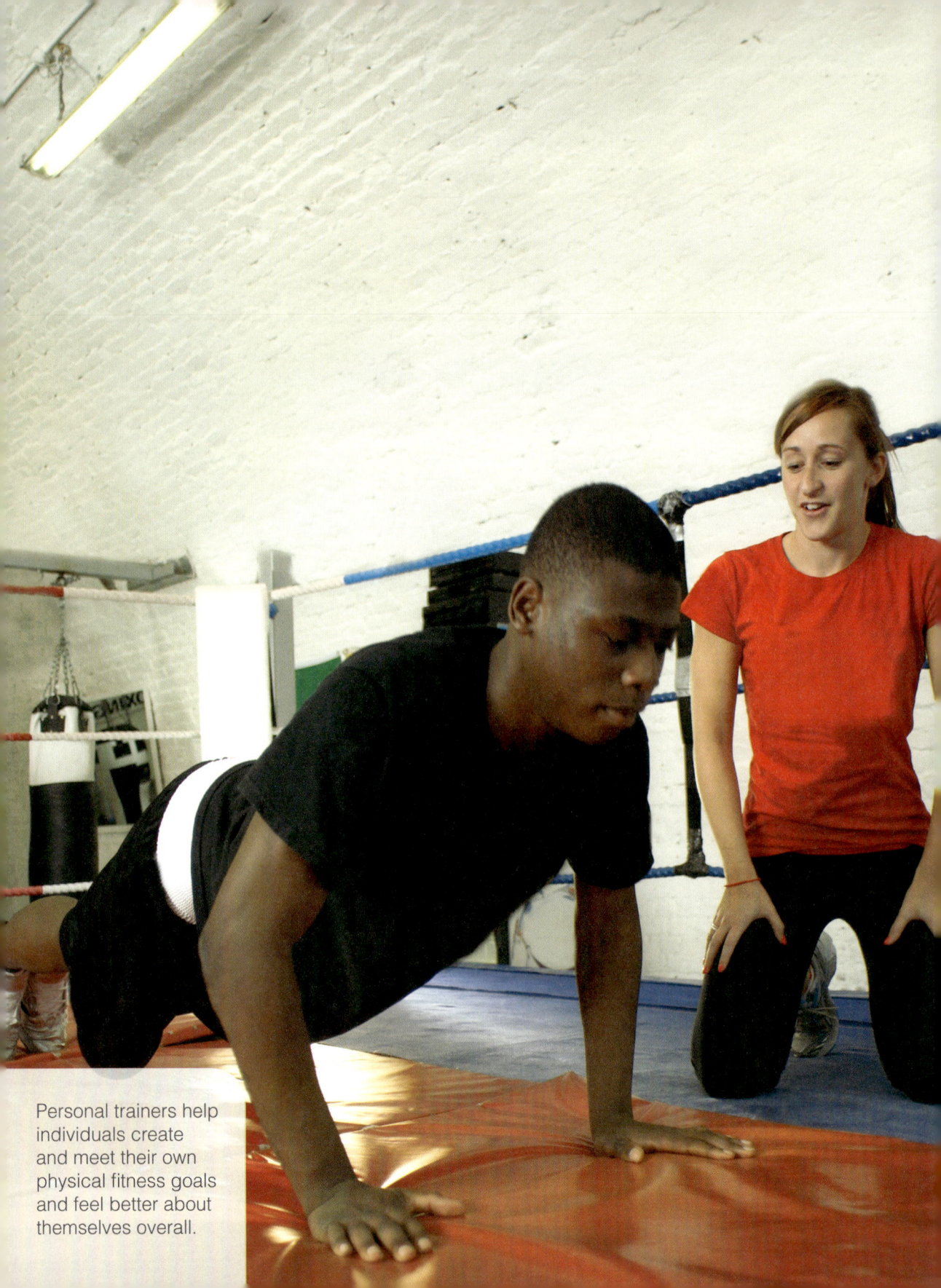

Working with Individuals

work from their homes, from offices, or from a gym. There is no official accreditation process, so an individual trainer is free to focus on different aspects of the exercise program.

A volunteer or an intern for a personal trainer might work in a gym, in a home office, or at clients' homes. Since the trainer is dedicated to improving a person's health, most have a wide variety of knowledge about nutrition, exercise, and the body. So an intern or volunteer can learn a lot about athletics from a different perspective. Interns or volunteers can expect to assist in administering general fitness and wellness tests, like measuring a person's pulse after running in place and recording results. Volunteers or interns may also demonstrate proper exercise methods.

Individual Lessons

Coaches often offer individual lessons to people who wish to improve particular skills in private. This allows for one-on-one training and direction in a sport. Unlike a personal trainer, the coach is generally not trying to figure out an entire exercise regiment for the person. If a person wants to practice throwing fastballs, learn how to better putt, or perfect form on a sprint, individual coaches could help.

A volunteer or intern to a coach giving individual lessons might help keep track of progress made, demonstrate particular moves, and serve as an opposing player when necessary.

Therapy Through Sports

Athletes know that having an injury can take a toll on a person—but therapy through sports can be both physically and emotionally healing.

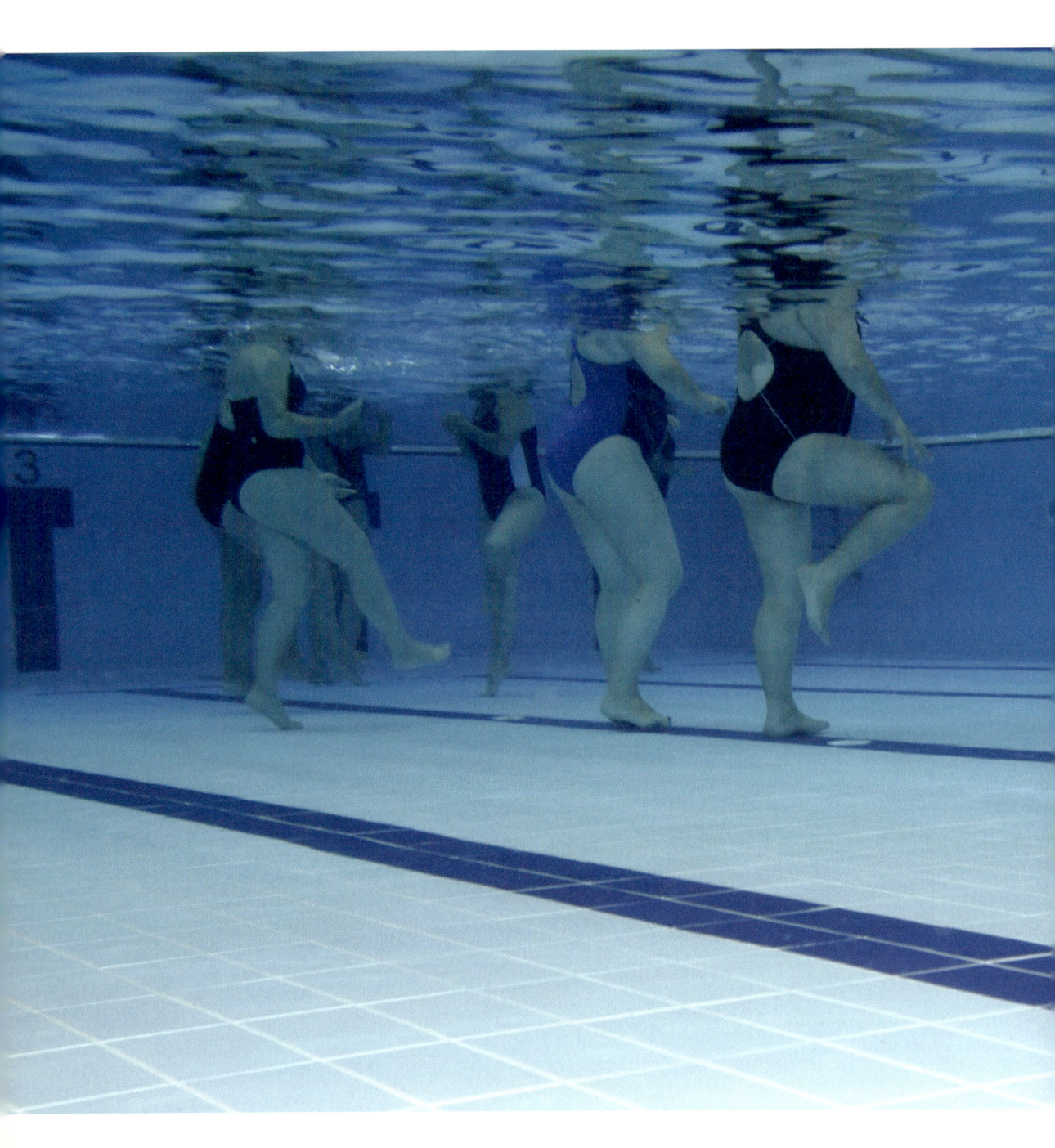

internship & volunteer opportunities for people who love movement

Physical therapy may appeal to individuals interested in helping others reach their peak performance.

Working with Individuals

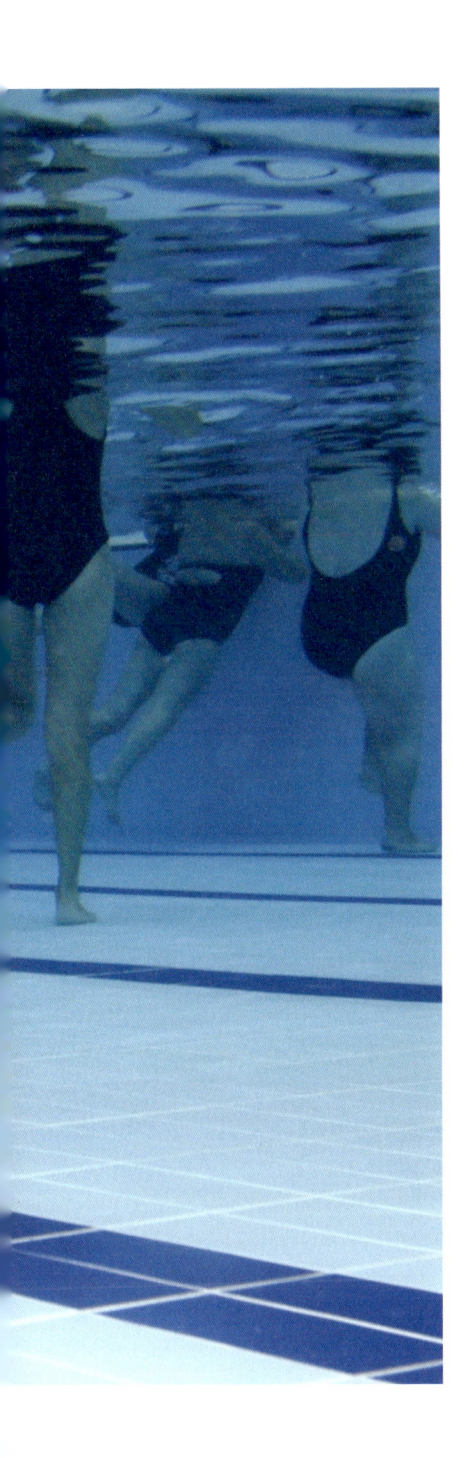

When a person has an injury that makes it uncomfortable to stand on hard surfaces for a long amount of time, land-based therapies are not very effective. Sometimes doctors may recommend aquatic therapies, which are exercises performed in a pool. This allows patients to move and get necessary exercise without as much pain because there is less joint pressure. An aquatic therapist creates a plan and guides patients through workouts, attempting to relieve pain and work muscles.

As an intern or volunteer to an aquatic therapist, you may be asked to help perform assessment tests, record data, and observe a patient's range of motion to determine the effectiveness of the therapy.

Horse therapy is another common way that sports are reported to have positive effects on a person's well-being. Some doctors and scientists claim that teaching a person with physical or cognitive disabilities to ride a horse not only improves physical fitness but also provides companionship and promotes compassionate behavior. Horse therapy is very active, involving not

internship & volunteer opportunities for people who love movement

Horse Therapy

In addition to helping people with physical or cognitive disorders, some experts say that horse therapy can also be helpful to people with behavioral or psychological problems. Part of that, they claim, is trust. Kathy Krupa is the founder of HorseTime, Inc., which pairs young people with psychiatric and emotional problems with horses. In an article in the *New York Times*, Krupa said that it is successful because "a horse couldn't care less if someone has been in jail or has a learning disability. They only judge you by how you are at the moment."

just grooming and basic riding but expanding to activities such as interactive vaulting, which the Professional Association of Therapeutic Horsemanship International describes as "gymnastics on horseback."

For someone who loves riding and wants to help others, volunteering or interning with horse therapy could be a great fit. An intern or volunteer would work with patients both in early stages as they get used to the animal, and then later on as they learn to ride and perform more difficult tricks and maneuvers. Interns or volunteers would model and assist patients with meeting, grooming, and riding the horse.

Working with Individuals

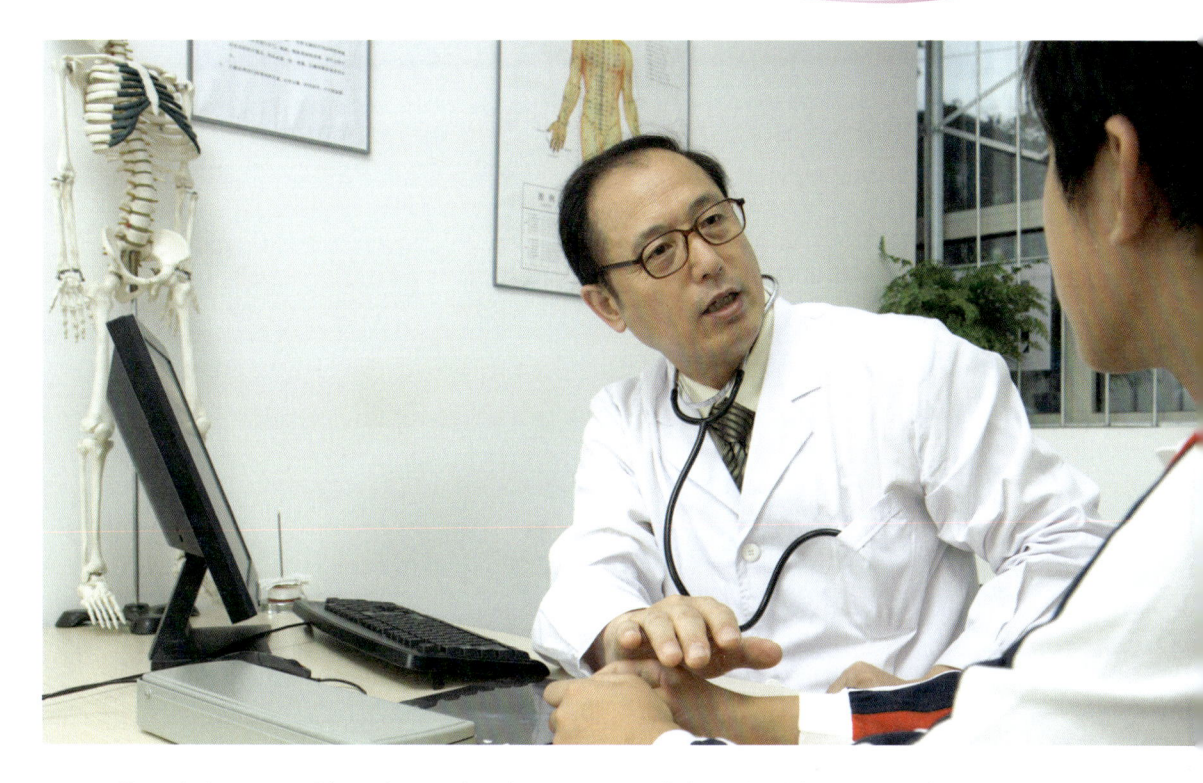

People interested in volunteering in sports medicine should talk to professionals in the field to get an idea of what opportunities exist.

Where to Look

Gyms often offer personal trainer services, so ask someone there about the best way to go about volunteering, or look online to find recommendations of good trainers in your area. To find a sports therapist, call a doctor and ask for a recommendation of someone to meet, or ask a coach if he or she knows someone to talk to. For individual lessons, watch for advertisements in newspapers, online, or flyers around town, and ask your family and friends if they know anyone.

Chapter Six

PERFORMING ARTS

Hamming it up onstage can be just as fun as running down the court—and be just as athletic, too! For young people who do not mind a bit of attention and like a lot of activity, the performing world has a lot to offer an intern or volunteer. Although other employees may already have filled the main performance roles, an intern or volunteer might be able to take on a smaller role or serve as an understudy, or a backup in case the main performer cannot fulfill his or her role at a given performance. The performance world is bustling with activity on and off the stage.

The Circus

When most people think of circuses, large-scale, three-ring traveling productions with exotic animals come to mind. This type of circus might offer volunteer or internship opportunities for young people, but young people

Performing Arts

should also consider more performance-based productions. The popular Cirque de Soleil, for example, describes itself as a combination of circus arts and street performances, and an active young person who likes to perform might be able to take the spotlight in an unusual way at such an organization.

Clowns are a popular part of most circuses. Despite the ploy of clowns being clumsy, playing this part may actually require quite a bit of coordination. Juggling, dancing, and tumbling are all common clown tricks. At some performances, clowns might spend the whole show on their feet, walking through the crowd and providing sideline entertainment. Interns or volunteers who enjoy making jokes and are outgoing may have an extra advantage in this role.

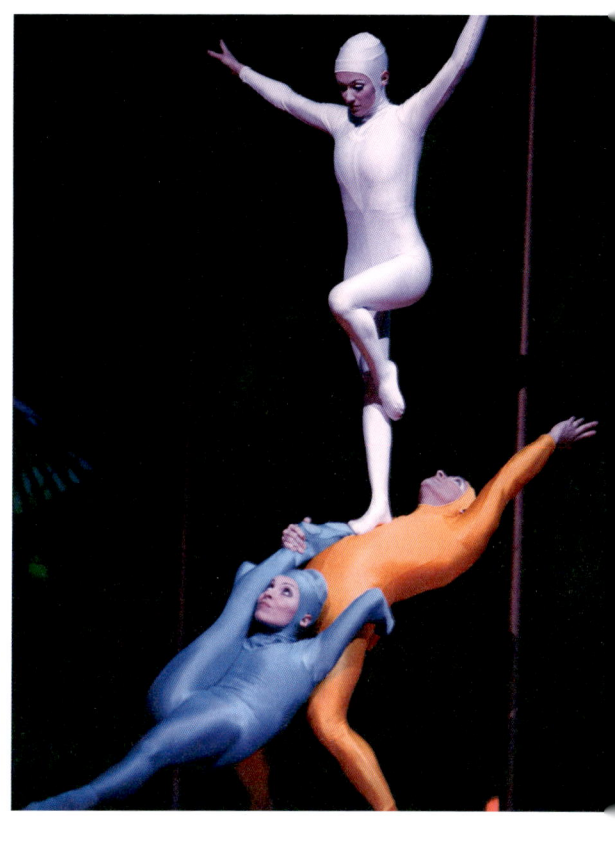

Being onstage can be a physically strenuous, yet exhilarating, experience, especially for people who perform acrobatics.

Acrobatics is another area in which an active young person might wish to participate in the circus. Many circus performers engage in some sort of acrobatic activity. Some perform playful dances and basic tumbles on the floor. Others engage in more dramatic tricks involving high-wire tightrope walking or elaborate trapeze work. Many acrobats who perform on these advanced

internship & volunteer opportunities for people who love movement

Working Onstage and Behind the Scenes

Although there are many opportunities for volunteering or interning onstage, do not forget about backstage, either. Building and moving sets are two ways that an athletic young person who loves the theater but does not want to be in the spotlight can participate in a performance.

Depending on the theater and on the performance, working on a play can be a very active role. Acting involves more than just standing in one place. Actors must move across the stage in a way that emphasizes their characters' words, actions, and emotions. If a play is a musical, it may even involve dancing. Many musicals involve larger groups of actors who make up a chorus, or a group of people meant to symbolize a crowd. An intern or volunteer in the theater might make his or her way onstage in one of these roles.

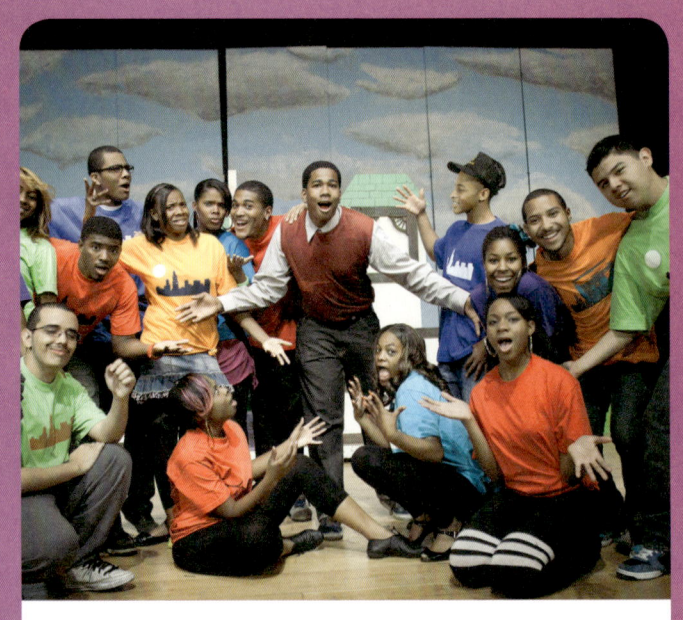

It takes a whole cast and crew of people to put on a play, and many of the roles require physical activity.

Performing Arts

levels have spent years training as gymnasts or have taken specialized classes. If you have previous experience with this sort of gymnastics, then you might have more of an opportunity to participate in the performance in a hands-on way.

Dance Troupes

Dance troupes are groups of dancers who perform together. Many dance troupes are composed of professional dancers. For this reason, it can be harder for an intern or volunteer with a dance

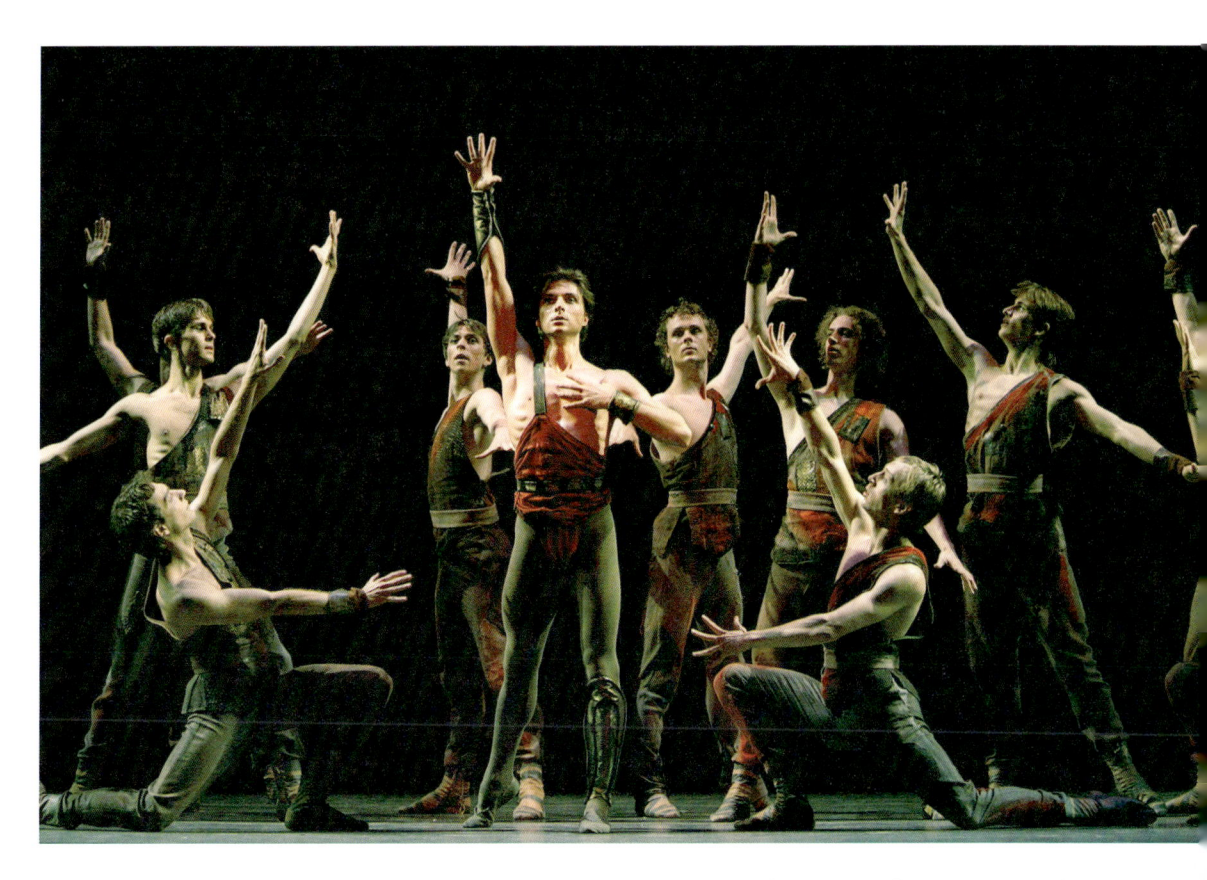

Dancers aren't the only ones moving about during a performance. Stagehands, often volunteers, move around just as much behind the scenes.

troupe to break into a main role on the stage—though as with theater, a volunteer or intern might fill an understudy or chorus role. But as with dance classes, an informed intern or volunteer can provide valuable feedback by watching the dancers carefully to make sure that everyone is in step and pointing out to the choreographer or director areas that need improvement. In a less formal dance troupe, a volunteer or intern might take on the role of helping with choreography as well.

Where to Look

Watch the pages of local newspapers and magazines for listings and reviews of upcoming performances, and call the organizing groups. Ask drama teachers at your school if they can recommend someone to talk to.

Chapter Seven

TOURISM AND RECREATION

Few people are as active as out-of-town visitors and vacationers, and many businesses exist to provide a variety of entertainment options for them. For an active young person, these businesses might offer the perfect volunteering or internship opportunity.

In the Water

In any area where there is water, there are probably a variety of businesses or organizations dedicated to water recreation. Some may require greater skills and previous knowledge than others; operating a rowboat might be easier than commanding a sailboat. But no matter what option you are interested in, it is important to be a strong swimmer—although if you are boating, hopefully you will not spend too much time actually in the water!

Boating is a popular tourist activity. There are many different types; sailing, kayaking, canoeing, and white-water

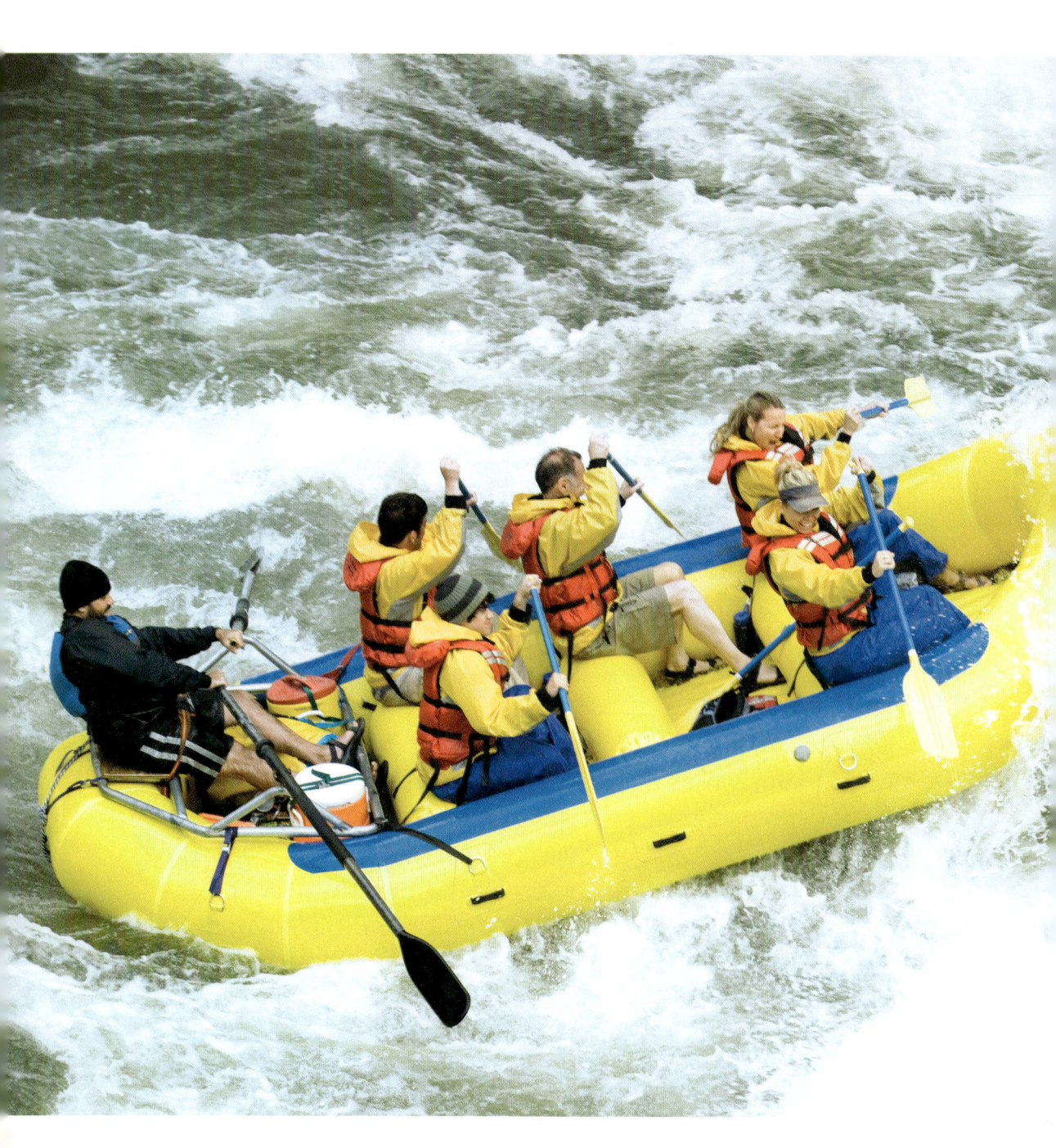

internship & volunteer opportunities for people who love movement

Rafting is a popular vacation activity, and tour companies often need help making sure people can enjoy the experience safely.

Tourism and Recreation

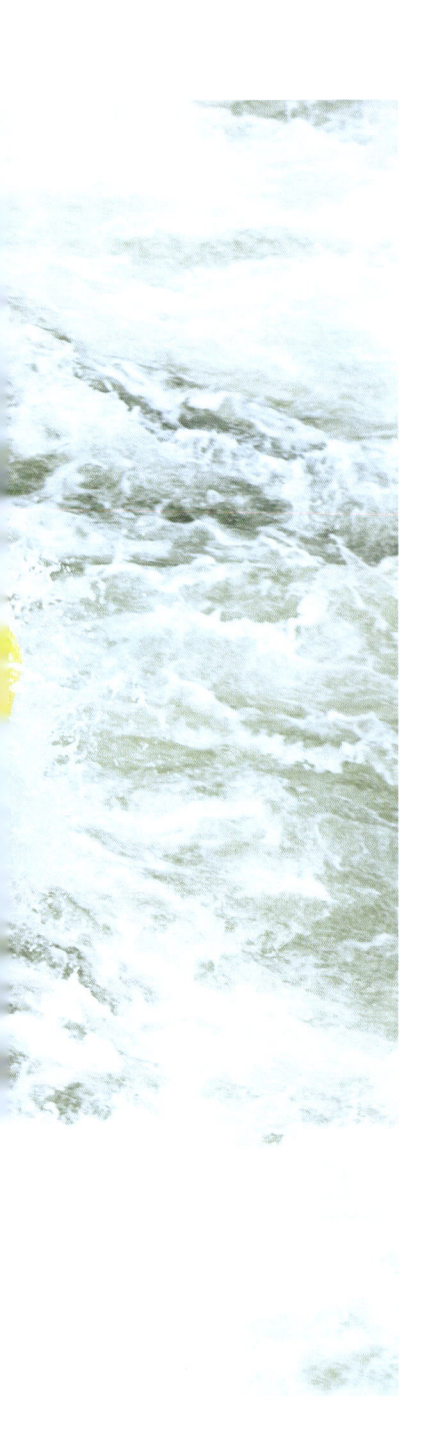

rafting are some of the most popular ones. Businesses based around boating might offer lessons, rides, or water tours of an area. A business that charges people for its services may have stricter requirements for its volunteers or interns who want to work hands-on with boating trips. Interns or volunteers for this type of organization need to demonstrate that they are skilled at directing the boat as well as excellent swimmers. Depending on the state and the type of boating, a person who leads trips may also be required to have a water license. Interns or volunteers for these businesses may help with trips if they meet the requirements. Otherwise, they might help out more with the behind-the-scenes work of running a business.

Some boating organizations offer free lessons to members of the community. They do this because they want others to learn to love the sport and to appreciate and protect the water. This is usually done for a type of boating that can be taught easily, like kayaking, canoeing, and paddle boating, because participants will have varying levels of skills. For this same reason, it is also easier for someone who does not have a lot of previous knowledge to work with these groups. With a little bit of practice and guidance, an intern or volunteer might develop his or her own skills enough to start demonstrating to others strokes and other boating methods. These free lessons can be short and designed just to introduce someone to the basics of boating.

Other times, organizations will lead longer tours, intending to show off the scenery or demonstrate a point about the area's ecology. Interns or volunteers on one of these trips might need to know more about where they are traveling and why. They might be asked to either narrate the trip, explaining the history of their surroundings, or answer questions that participants have. A volunteer or intern for this type of organization might also work with publicizing the lessons, finding sponsors to help cover the costs of the lessons, and organizing the participants.

Scuba diving and snorkeling are two other popular water activities that offer opportunities for young people. Many businesses offer lessons and trips. Depending on the state, a license and a training course may be required before becoming officially registered as a snorkeler or diver, and additional training may be necessary before being able to teach or assist with lessons.

For those who prefer to stay in the sun and make their way into water only occasionally, volunteering or interning as a lifeguard might be the best bet. Many nonprofit organizations run camps or programs that include swimming, and they need strong swimmers with a sharp eye to make sure everyone is staying safe on the beach or at the pool. Lifeguarding often requires passing a course and obtaining CPR certification. Colleges and community centers in your area might offer these courses.

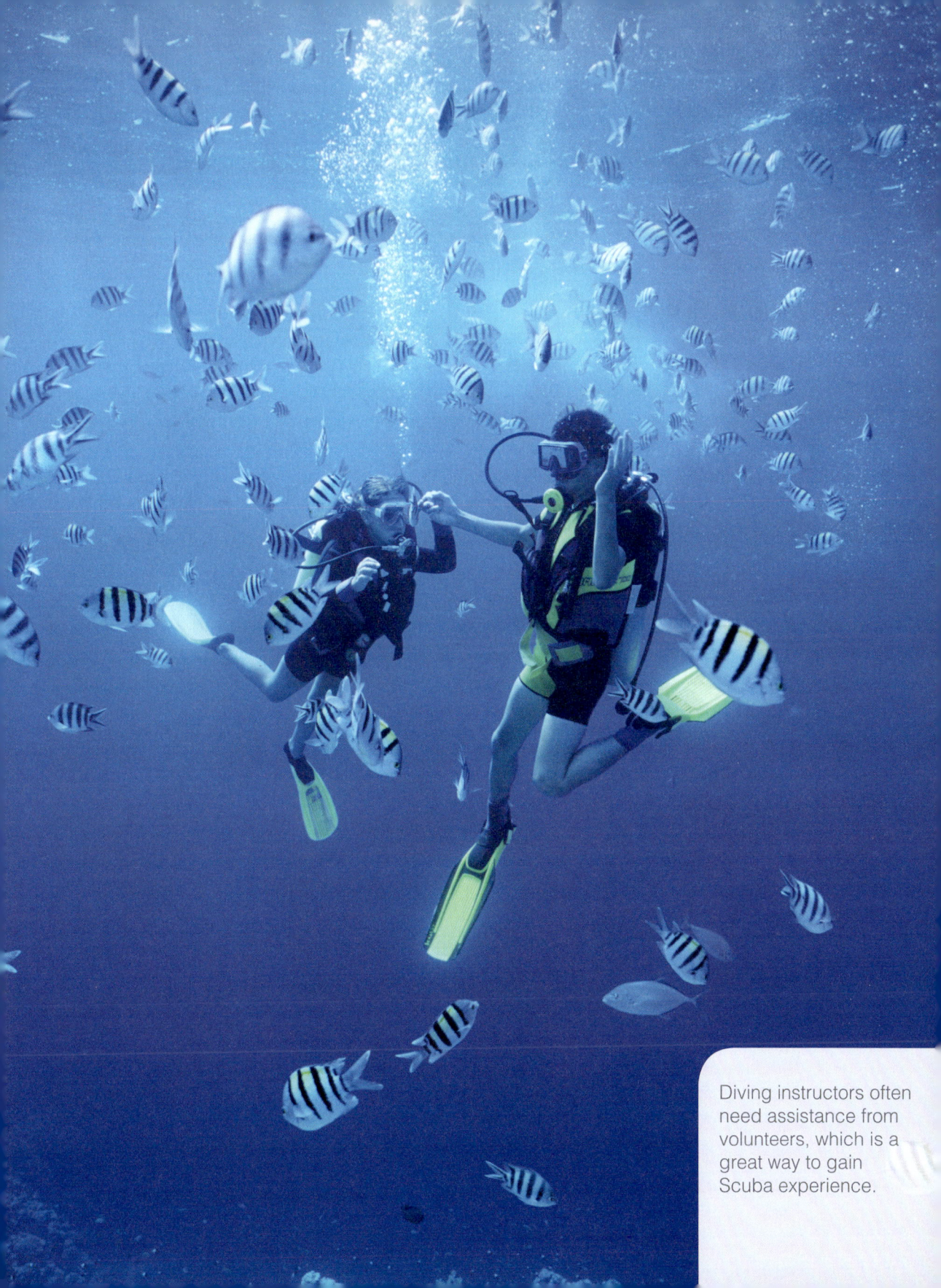

Diving instructors often need assistance from volunteers, which is a great way to gain Scuba experience.

internship & volunteer opportunities for people who love movement

On Land

For those who prefer to explore the woods rather than the water, working in a park might be a better option. According to the National Park Service, there are 397 designated national parks in the United States. These include a range of land types, from forests to deserts. There are a number of other sites, not officially designated, that offer the same outdoor setting. Interns might work

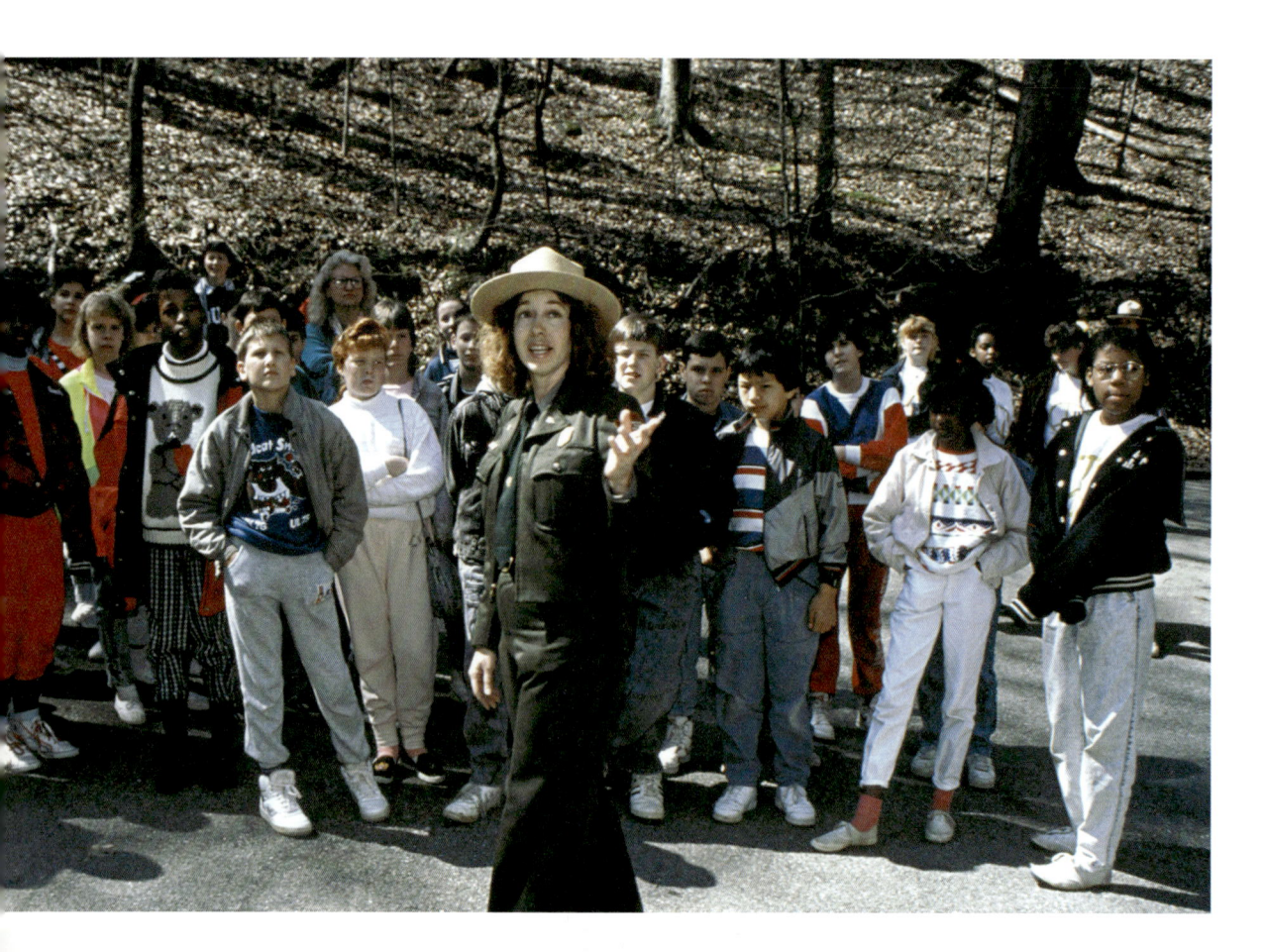

Leading a tour of a national park requires physical fitness and a variety of historical and geographic knowledge.

closely with a park ranger, leading hikes, clearing trails, answering questions, and making sure that everything is in order and safe for the many visitors.

Snow lovers have plenty of options for interning and volunteering, too. Skilled skiers and snowboarders might intern at a ski slope, where people ranging from complete beginners to absolute pros visit to take a ride down the hills. Beginners require extra lessons and help, so an intern who knows a lot about the sport might assist with a class that teach the basics, including demonstrating how to position the body, how to stop, and how to safely fall. A skilled volunteer might find an outdoor fair or fund-raiser and offer to demonstrate there.

National Parks

Yellowstone National Park was the first ever established national park in 1872. In the years since, the government has added to the list when it determines that the natural existence of an area should be protected from human development. These areas are often beautiful, but in order to be named a national park, scientists must also provide information about the ecological life of an area and why it must be protected. For young people who love the environment as well as staying active, interning or volunteering at a national park is a great way to combine interests and skills.

internship & volunteer opportunities for people who love movement

Where to Look

Young people interested in working with tourism businesses should see if their towns have a chamber of commerce, which is an organization that links local companies, and ask for a copy of the directory listing its member companies. They can then contact businesses that fit what they are looking for. Look up books or Web sites that list recommended activities for visitors, and check out the companies associated with them.

For young people who would like to volunteer, check out local newspapers and magazines to find listings of upcoming events. If there is an event that matches with your skills and needs, contact the organizer and ask if anyone needs help.

In a small town, there might not be as many options for recreational and tourism jobs. If you find that your town does not offer the type of experience you are looking for, think about your family and friends who live in other places. Is there somewhere you could stay for a couple of weeks while trying out one of these experiences?

Chapter Eight
MAKING THE MOST OF YOUR EXPERIENCE

So you have landed your dream internship or volunteer position—now what? You put in a lot of work and did your research, and it has paid off. But how can you be sure that your internship or volunteer experience is everything it should be?

Setting Goals and Expectations

When you start your experience, it may become clear to you that there is a particular person you go to when you have questions or need help. This person is your supervisor. He or she may also take on the form of a career mentor, or a person who guides and advises you in your professional development. It is a good idea to talk to this person early on about what his or her expectations for you are. How long will your experience last? How often will you work? Is there something specific that you should accomplish in your time? If you are doing an internship

Professional Behavior

Different organizations have different cultures. Since your opportunity may be more athletics-based, your professional attire is probably a bit different than that of someone who works in a traditional office. You will want to wear something that is appropriate for the hours at the gym and on the field. But this does not mean that professional behavior is any less important.

In athletics, competition can get heated, but when you are on the professional side, keep your temper in check and always be a good sport. Be polite and respectful of supervisors, coworkers, and people you come into contact with.

Arrive on time and focus completely on work each day when you arrive. Put away your cell phone, iPod, and books to make it clear that you are not distracted.

Keep a positive outlook, even if you are doing some tasks that you do not like—everyone has to do some of these chores. But if after a while you find that you are not ever doing the type of work you are interested in, it might be time to talk to your supervisor.

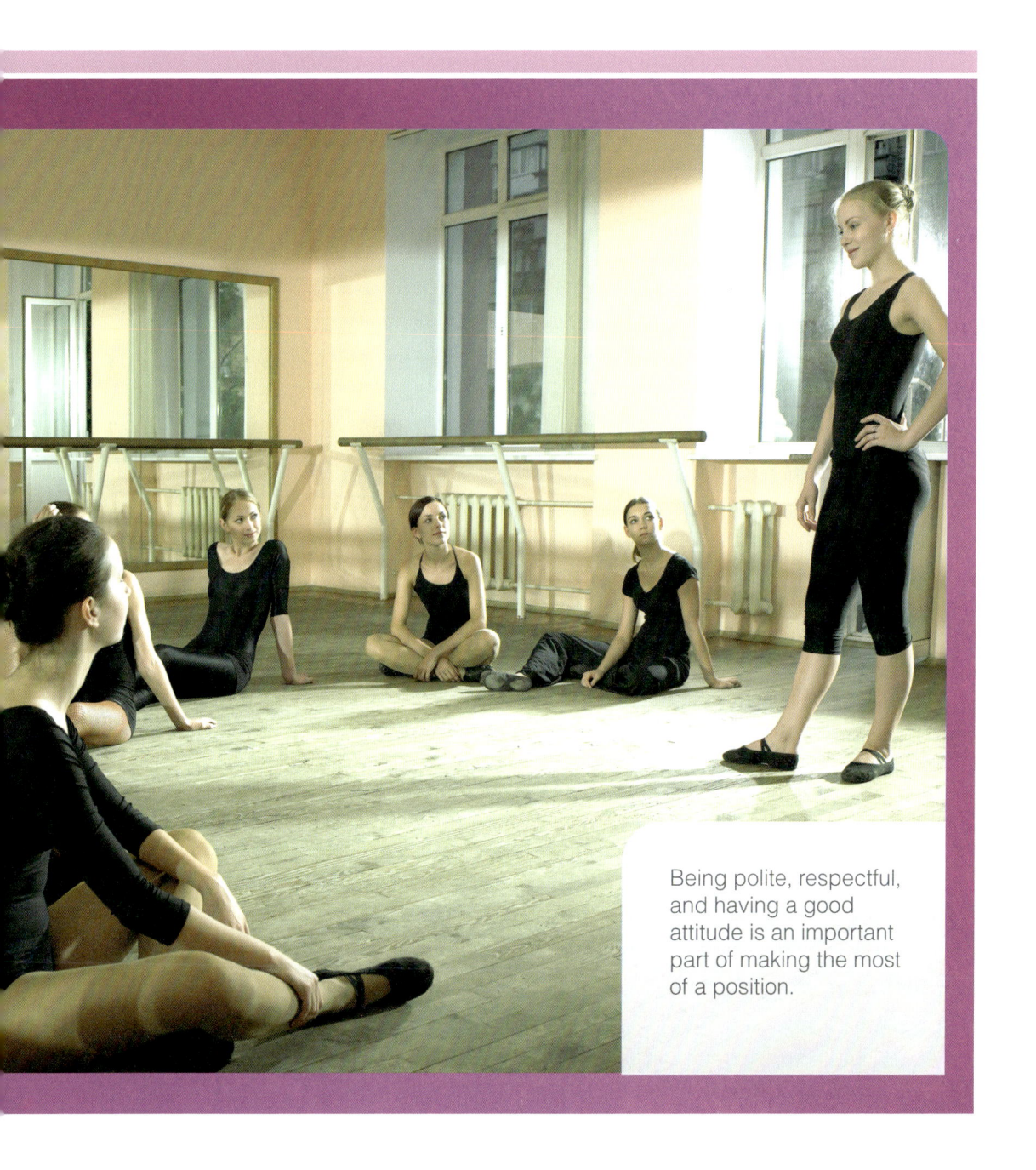

Making the Most of Your Experience

Being polite, respectful, and having a good attitude is an important part of making the most of a position.

internship & volunteer opportunities for people who love movement

for academic credit, your course work may require a particular learning agreement to be signed by both you and your supervisor outlining these rules and expectations.

In some less formal internship or volunteer situations, you may not have such a structured setting to ask these questions. Especially in instances where you are working with a smaller organization or the organization has not had interns or volunteers before you, you and your supervisor may be figuring out the structure of your experience as you go. In these instances, it is helpful to do this reflection yourself. What are you hoping to get out of this experience? How will you know you are achieving this? Setting goals for yourself will help you maintain focus and make sure that you are making the most of your time.

Finding Opportunities for New Responsibilities

When you have been at your internship or volunteer opportunity for a while and have found that your responsibilities are not increasing, you might try to find new ways to help at the same organization or company.

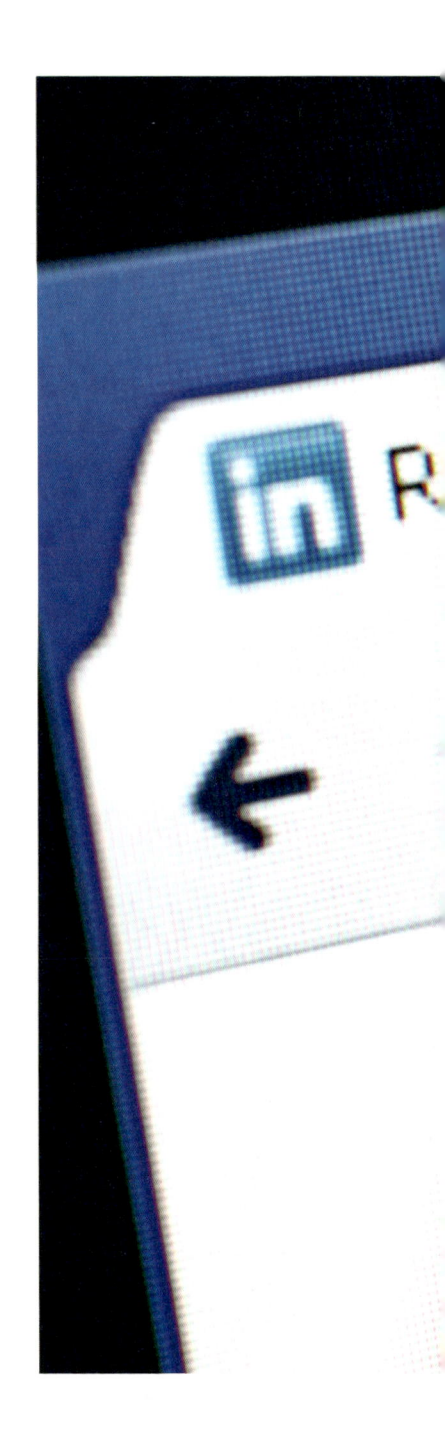

Making the Most of Your Experience

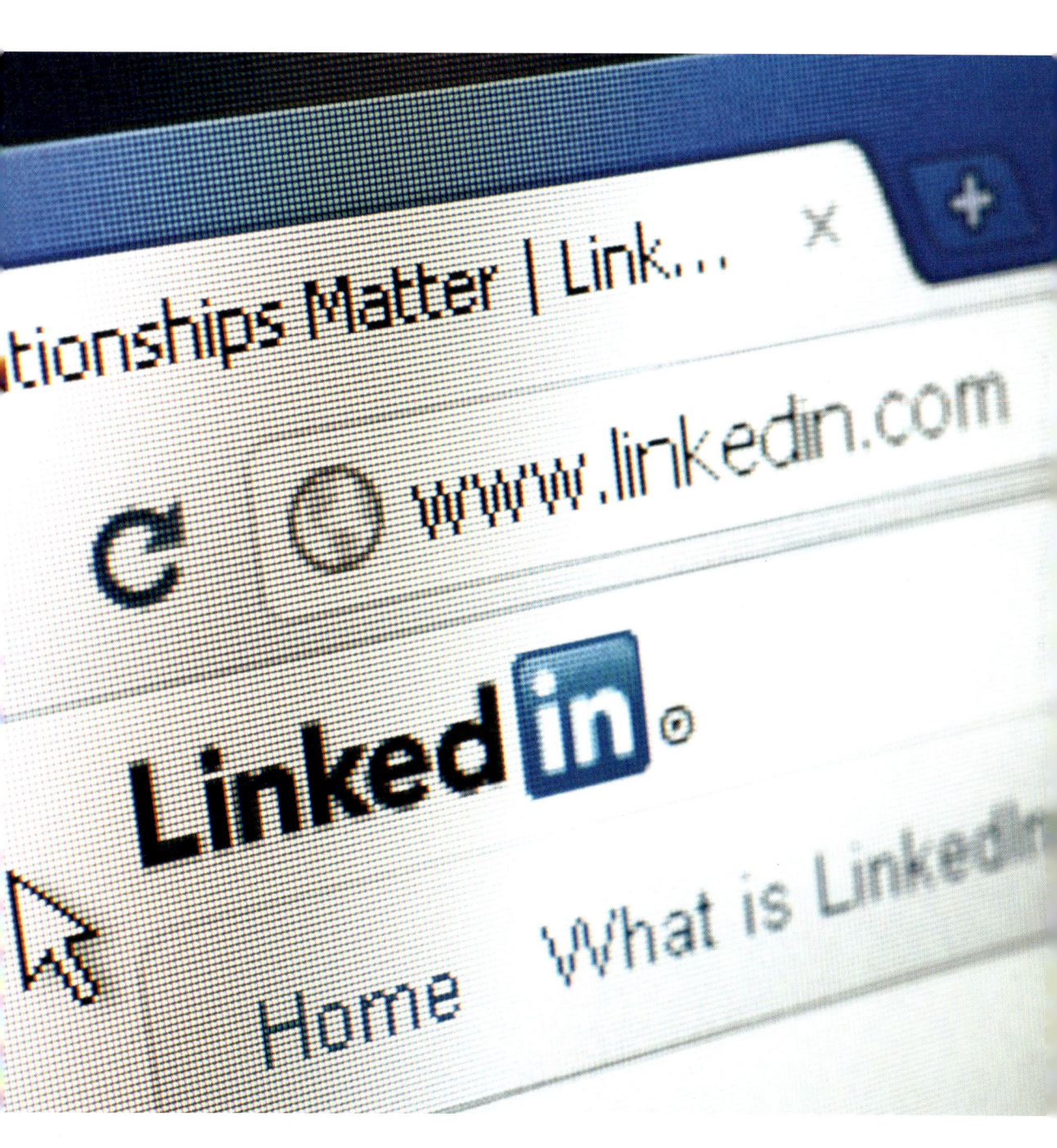

Don't forget to search for and stay in touch with professional connections using career networking sites such as LinkedIn (http://www.linkedin.com).

First, take an honest assessment of the situation. Are the tasks you are more interested in things that you know how to do or could easily be trained in? Are they tasks that an organization is able to hand over to an intern or volunteer? Sometimes for professional reasons, an employee may be required to do particular work even if an intern or volunteer is capable of taking it on. If a task is not something that you can do yet, then watch other employees carefully and learn as much as you can from that.

If you do not have a lot to do, pay attention to your surroundings and observe other people as they work. Is there one person who is always overwhelmed? If so, it may be a better use of your, and the organization's, time to help that person. Maybe the fifth-grade soccer team at the YMCA does not need so much help, but the first-grade team could use an extra hand.

Above all, talk to your supervisor about the situation. You are helping him or her out, but your supervisor wants you to benefit from your experience, too. Together, figure out if there is a new way that you can get the experience you are looking for.

Keeping Track of Your Achievements

After you finish volunteering or interning each day, take mental inventory of what you have achieved. If you prefer, keep track of it in a journal or on a chart. It does not have to be extensive, but after you have been working toward a goal for a while, it can be hard to remember how far you have come. Just thinking about your work each day will help you to maintain focus on your goal, and it will help you be better able to articulate your achievements in the future.

Making the Most of Your Experience

When it is time for you to find a new experience, you want to be able to showcase everything you have achieved. You can do this by creating specific résumé point descriptions and a portfolio. For the résumé point descriptions, use specific facts and numbers to show off just how much you have achieved (e.g., served as assistant coach for regional champion team of eighteen fifth graders). Keep copies of any media coverage, and take photographs (if children are involved, get parents' permission first). Combine this information in a professional-looking binder or on a Web site. Now you have not only a valuable job-searching resource demonstrating your accomplishments, but you also have a scrapbook.

Parting Professionally

When you have reached the end of your volunteer or internship opportunity, be sure to thank everyone who helped you along the way. Send notes to anyone who put you in contact with the organization. Thank in person everyone whom you worked with, and follow up with a note to your supervisor. Ask for a letter of recommendation, and do not forget to show it off in your next interview. Connect with anyone who is on professional networking sites such as LinkedIn—but hold back on less formal Facebook requests. Keep in touch and let your supervisor know what you are up to, especially if you find a new position.

Glossary

career field An area of job specialization that is often practiced over many years.

cover letter A note introducing a job candidate's résumé and providing additional information about his or her qualifications.

extrovert A person who enjoys and is energized by interactions with other people.

informational interview A meeting to share knowledge of a particular career field.

internship An entry-level training position, often open to high school and college students who are looking to learn more about a particular career field.

interview A meeting to determine if a person is the best fit for an open position.

introvert A person who enjoys and is energized by being alone.

jujitsu A form of martial arts that originated in Japan and emphasizes hand movement and throwing.

LinkedIn A social networking Web site where a person lists relevant experiences and can make professional connections.

mentor A person who provides guidance and advice on career goals and decisions.

nonprofit organization An organization, often focused on charity, that does not profit financially from its work.

Pilates A form of exercise that emphasizes building core muscles.

Glossary

portfolio A collection of materials and samples, either online or hard copy, that demonstrates the range of a person's, usually artistic, work.

résumé A listing of relevant work, academic, and volunteer experiences and achievements.

tae kwon do A form of martial arts that originated in Korea and emphasizes leg movement and kicking.

understudy In a performance, the person who fills in for a role if its primary actor or performer is unable to.

volunteer A person who offers to help an organization or company without pay.

yoga A form of exercise that historically combines spiritual well-being with physical fitness.

For More Information

Congressional Youth Leadership Council
1919 Gallows Road, Suite 700
Vienna, VA 22182
Web site: http://www.cylc.org
The Congressional Youth Leadership Council (CYLC) is a program that nurtures young people who exhibit academic achievement and leadership skills, including in the business realm.

Junior Achievement
One Education Way
Colorado Springs, CO 8090
(719) 540-8000
Web site: http://www.ja.org
Junior Achievement is an organization that teaches teens skills essential to success in the business world.

National Collegiate Athletic Association
700 W. Washington Street
P.O. Box 6222
Indianapolis, IN 46206-6222
(317) 917-6222
Web site: http://www.ncaa.org
The National Collegiate Athletic Association creates and enforces standards in college athletics.

For More Information

National Park Service
1849 C Street NW
Washington, DC 2024
(202) 208-3818
Web site: http://www.nps.gov
The National Park Service oversees the upkeep of and coordinates volunteers and employees for all national parks in the United States.

Office of Travel & Tourism Industries
14th & Constitution Avenue NW
Washington, DC 20230
Web site: http://tinet.ita.doc.gov
The Office of Travel & Tourism Industries is a U.S. government agency that provides statistical information and research on domestic tourism.

Web Sites

Due to the changing nature of Internet links, Rosen Publishing has developed an online list of Web sites related to the subject of this book. This site is updated regularly. Please use this link to access the list:

http://www.rosenlinks.com/FID/Mov

For Further Reading

Allen, Jeffrey G. *Instant Interviews: 101 Ways to Get the Best Job of Your Life.* Hoboken, NJ: Wiley, 2009.

Camenson, Blythe. *Careers for Aquatic Types & Others Who Want to Make a Splash.* 2nd ed. New York, NY: McGraw-Hill, 2008.

Eikleberry, Carol. *The Career Guide for Creative and Unconventional People.* 3rd ed. Berkeley, CA: Ten Speed Press, 2007.

Horn, Geoffrey M. *Sports Therapist.* Pleasantville, NY: Gareth Stevens, 2009.

Kenworthy, Kate, and Stephen A. Rodrigues. *The Everything Guide to Being a Personal Trainer: All You Need to Get Started on a Career in Fitness.* Avon, MA: Adams Media, 2007.

Landes, Michael. *The Back Door Guide to Short-Term Job Adventures: Internships, Summer Jobs, Seasonal Work, Volunteer Vacations, and Transitions Abroad.* 4th ed. Berkeley, CA: Ten Speed Press, 2005.

Lewis, Barbara A. *The Teen Guide to Global Action: How to Connect with Others (Near & Far) to Create Social Change.* Minneapolis, MN: Free Spirit Publishing, 2008.

Liptak, John J. *Career Quizzes: 12 Tests to Help You Discover and Develop Your Dream Career.* Indianapolis, IN: JIST Works, 2008.

Lore, Nicholas, and Anthony Spadafore. *Now What?: The Young Person's Guide to Choosing the Perfect Career.* New York, NY: Simon & Schuster, 2008.

Tieger, Paul D., and Barbara Tieger. *Do What You Are: Discover the Perfect Career for You Through the Secrets of Personality Type.* 4th ed. New York, NY: Little, Brown and Co., 2007.

Waldman, Joshua. *Job Searching with Social Media for Dummies.* Hoboken, NJ: Wiley, 2011.

Wong, Glenn M. *The Comprehensive Guide to Careers in Sports.* 2nd ed. Burlington, MA: Jones & Bartlett Learning, 2012.

Yate, Martin John. *Knock 'Em Dead Cover Letters: The Strategies and Samples You Need to Get the Job You Want.* 9th ed. Avon, MA: Adams Media, 2010.

Bibliography

Berger, Sandra L. *The Ultimate Guide to Summer Opportunities for Teens: 200 Programs That Prepare You for College Success.* Waco, TX: Prufrock Press, 2008.

Bolles, Richard Nelson. *What Color Is Your Parachute?: A Practical Manual for Job-Hunters and Career-Changers.* 40th Anniversary ed. Berkeley, CA: Ten Speed, 2011.

Flender, Nicole. *Cool Careers Without College For People Who Love Movement.* New York, NY: Rosen Publishing, 2002.

Heitzmann, William Ray. *Careers for Sports Nuts & Other Athletic Types.* 3rd ed. Chicago, IL: VGM Career Books, 2004.

Johnson, Nathan. *Martial Arts for the Mind: Essential Tips, Drills, and Combat Techniques.* Broomall, PA: Mason Crest, 2005.

Loveland, Elaina C. *Creative Careers: Paths for Aspiring Actors, Artists, Dancers, Musicians and Writers.* 2nd ed. Belmont, CA: Supercollege, 2009.

Petitpas, Albert J. *Athlete's Guide to Career Planning.* Champaign, IL: Human Kinetics, 1997.

Silas, Elizabeth, and Diane Goodney. *Yoga.* New York, NY: Franklin Watts, 2003.

Troutman, Kathryn K. *Creating Your High School Resume: A Step-by-Step Guide to Preparing an Effective Resume for Jobs, College, and Training Programs.* 2nd ed. Indianapolis: JIST Works, 2003.

Index

A

academic/school credit, getting, 7, 14, 68
achievements, keeping track of, 70–71
application process for positions, 20–22

B

books, for research, 15

C

circus, the, 52–55
coaching, 32–36, 45, 47, 51
cover letters, 27

D

dance, 40–42, 44
 troupes, 55–56

F

Facebook, 15, 25, 71

G

goals and expectations, setting, 65–68
guidance counselors, getting help from, 12–14, 15

H

horse therapy, 49–50

I

individuals, working with, 45–51
informational interviews, 18–19, 22–23
interests, researching your, 8–11
Internet, using for research, 15, 18
internships
 about, 6, 7
 brainstorming ideas for, 8–11, 15, 17, 18
 finding opportunities, 20–31
 parting from, 71
interviews, tips for, 30–31

L

LinkedIn, 17–18, 25, 71
local resources, 25–27

M

martial arts, 42–44

N

national parks, 62, 63

Index

P

Paterno, Joe, 34
performing arts, 52–56
personal connections, using, 22–23
personal training, 45–47, 51
Pilates, 40, 44
professional behavior, importance of, 66

R

responsibilities, taking on new, 68–70
résumés, 27, 71
   tips for, 28–29

S

school resources, 12–14, 22
social media/networking
   and finding opportunities, 23–25, 71
   using for research, 15–18
sports therapy, 47–50, 51
supervisor, talking to your, 65, 66, 70, 71

T

teaching, 37–44
tourism and recreation, 57–64
   on land, 62–63
   in the water, 57–60
Twitter, 15–17, 23

V

volunteering
   about, 5–6, 7
   brainstorming ideas for, 8–11, 15, 17, 18
   finding opportunities, 20–31
   parting from, 71

Y

yoga, 37–39, 40, 44

internship & volunteer opportunities for people who love movement

About the Author

Susan Dobinick lives in New York City and works in youth media.

Photo Credits

Cover © iStockphoto.com/Mikhail Zykov; pp. 4–5 iStockphoto/Thinkstock; p. 9 Yellow Dog Productions/The Image Bank/Getty Images; p. 10 David Oliver/Taxi/Getty Images; pp. 12–13 © Spencer Grant/PhotoEdit; pp. 16–17 Brendan O'Sullivan/Photolibrary/Getty Images; p. 21 Comstock Images/Thinkstock; pp. 24–25 Yuri Arcurs/Shutterstock.com; p. 26 Stephen Mcsweeney/Shutterstock.com; pp. 29, 48–49 Hemera/Thinkstock; p. 30 Marilyn Angel Wynn/Nativestock/Getty Images; p. 33 Chuck Solomon/Sports Illustrated/Getty Images; p. 35 oliveromg/Shutterstock.com; p. 39 Getty Images/Digital Vision/ Thinkstock; pp. 40–41 Image Source/Getty Images; p. 43 © iStockphoto.com/kzenon; p. 46 Peter Muller/Cultura/Getty Images; p. 51 blue jean images/Getty Images; p. 53 Greetsia Tent/WireImage/Getty Images; p. 54 Hill Street Studios/Blend Images/ Getty Images; p. 55 Paul Hawthorne/Getty Images; pp. 58–59 Erik Isakson/Getty Images; p. 61 Jeff Rotman/The Image Bank/Getty Images; p. 62 Jeff Greenberg/Peter Arnold/Getty Images; pp. 66–67 Hans Neleman/Taxi/Getty Images; pp. 68–69 © iStockphoto.com/Günay Mutlu.

Designer: Michael Moy; Editor: Nicholas Croce;
Photo Researcher: Marty Levick